ME? I'M STILL HERE

Beating cancer isn't brave. It's survival.

TANIA BOND

Bloomington, IN 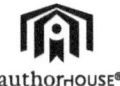 Milton Keynes, UK

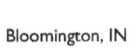

AuthorHouse™
1663 Liberty Drive, Suite 200
Bloomington, IN 47403
www.authorhouse.com
Phone: 1-800-839-8640

AuthorHouse™ UK Ltd.
500 Avebury Boulevard
Central Milton Keynes, MK9 2BE
www.authorhouse.co.uk
Phone: 08001974150

First published by AuthorHouse 1/30/2007

ISBN: 978-1-4259-7194-6 (sc)

Printed in the United States of America
Bloomington, Indiana

This book is printed on acid-free paper.

This book was written daily to help me through, and beat cancer. I hope that by making it into a book and having it published it will help someone as much as it did me.

Tania.

Table Of Contents

To my beautiful husband.
Thank you for being you, W.W.S.
I Love You. x

To my Dad.
Not gone, just borrowed. x

To Jake, Molly, Bill, Fred, John and Lucy.
I hope that this book makes what
happened easier to understand.
I love you all so very much.
Mum. x

To my mum, mum and dad.
Thank you for all your patience and time you
gave me, and a special thank you for
all the cuddles. x

Acknowledgements

I would like to thank all the staff at the Great Western Hospital, especially the nurses in Wren, Osprey and Beech ward.

All the people at the Churchill Hospital in the Radiology Department.

The oncologists based at the hospitals in Oxford especially the one that suggested that I have my book printed for a larger audience.

Also the wonderful people at the Priory Road Medical Centre.

In fact thank you everyone who has helped me through the last twenty four months.

Disclaimer.

―――◆◆◆―――

Everything that is in this book is my interpretation of events that took place during the time I was being treated for cancer.

Any medication or treatment I took or was given, was the most suitable for me. Everyone is an individual and therefore medication and treatment that works for one person may not work or suit another.

Symptoms and side-effects are also unique to everyone and need to be checked. My book is not a medical reference book, but my day to day diary, which I wanted to share.

Please do not self diagnose or use anything I did without consulting either your doctor, oncologists or someone who is a registered professional in their field.

Introduction

This is the day-to-day diary of me living with breast cancer.

There is nothing brave about "battling" cancer, you don't have a choice.

If you don't have the treatment you could die. It's as simple as that.

Soldiers that go to war are brave. They chose to go there, they chose to live or die.

Having Cancer doesn't give you a choice, but you have an inbuilt will to survive and the will to do anything to live.

There is nothing brave about having chemotherapy, it has to be done.

There was nothing brave about having my breasts removed. It had to be done.

I have to survive and live to a ripe old age.

I have met my hero, my sole mate and my lover in my beautiful husband.

There is too much love for it to end early.

I have six fantastic little people to nurture and help grow up into brilliant adults.

So having cancer isn't about being brave, it's just a blip in my life.

It's the strength builder, making me a stronger, tougher and a more determined person.

It's made me take everything life can throw at me, rather than just sitting and letting it pass me by.

But, yes it is very, very hard to get through!

Chapter I

———◆———

August

I finished feeding Freddy when he was nine months old.

I caught sight of myself in the mirror a couple of weeks later and thought that my boobs looked a bit sad and saggy.

It was while I was washing that I noticed that rather than them being all lumpy, they had become smooth apart from one small lump above my right nipple. I didn't think much about it, but I had a feeling in my tummy that it wasn't right.

I rang the doctor's surgery and was told that my own doctor was on holiday until next week, so I made an appointment to see her then.

September

September 2nd

I went to see the doctor and she examined me. Yes, there was a lump and because of my family history she was going to book me in to see a specialist at the hospital.

September 9th

My first appointment at the hospital. Steve came with me. We went into the breast care unit and waited. I was called through, they told me to go into the cubicles and take off my top and bra and put on a gown.

I did this and then went into another room where there must have been at least a dozen ladies waiting.

One lady was getting married on Saturday, another was complaining how bored she was and there was one old lady who had been there all day and had her shopping with her.

I was called into the examination room and told to lay down with my right arm above my head. A doctor came in and examined me. Yes, there was a lump. He used a scanner machine and looked at it again. He moved it up and down. The picture on the screen looked like one of those sand pictures. You couldn't make out the lump. It just looked like lots of layers, with one of them having an arc shape in it.

"We are going to take a sample," said the doctor. They sprayed some pink solution onto my breast and put in a needle. I made the mistake of looking at the doctor's face. He gritted his teeth as he took the sample.

"Better take another one." He said. Again he gritted his teeth. "Did that hurt?" He asked .

"If I had been my husband, you would have been on the floor by now." I replied.

He smiled and laughed nervously.

"We will make an appointment for you for next week to get the results." He said. "Oh, and before you go the surgeon would like to see you."

I waited outside and after a while I was called into another room where there was a smiley man sitting behind a desk, he was wearing a spotty bow-tie.

"Hello." he said. He talked over what had just been done and examined me again. I left after he said that he would see me again when I came back next week.

I went home quite happy. They didn't seem over concerned. It didn't look that nasty to me. That was a good sign. I thought that I would go back and they would say everything was fine.

September 17ᵗʰ

NIGHTMARE! My appointment was at 2:40pm. I was seem at 3:50pm. I took a deep breath and went in, again I was examined. I put my clothes back on.

"I'm sorry." said the surgeon with the bow-tie. "The results were not conclusive. We need to do a core biopsy. It's done under a local anaesthetic.""That's fine." I replied. I was told that I would be sent another appointment.

September 18th

HAPPY BIRTHDAY ASHLEY.

September 19th

HAPPY BIRTHDAY DAD!

September 22nd

I returned to the breast clinic and was asked to put on a gown and wait to be called in. It was a different doctor this time. In the room with him were two nurses, one of them was a student. He gave me loads of anaesthetic and then picked up a scalpel.

"Would you like me to hold your hand?" asked one of the nurses. "Was it that obvious?" I replied.

The doctor, two nurses and myself were chatting about everything and anything. The doctor was brilliant. He put me completely at ease. It was soon over and they patched me up. The nurse said she would see if the results could be rushed through so that I could be told at the end of the week rather than waiting another whole week.

I was given a cup of tea while the nurse sorted it out. Good news, they could do it, I would know the results on Friday.

September 24th

I was sitting in the waiting room when the surgeon with the bow-tie opened his door and looked out. He gave me eye contact but he did not smile. That was it! I knew then. I've got cancer. My stomach went heavy. Tears started to fall, I wasn't crying they just fell out. I was called in, "It's bad news I'm afraid Mrs Bond," he said, "you have breast cancer.""I know." I replied. He looked confused. "When you opened the door and saw me, you didn't smile." "Oh." He said."Right! So what are you going to do about it?" I said. There were several choices. I could just have the lump removed, have the whole breast removed or have it removed and then rebuilt with an implant.

I asked to have them both removed, as he told me that there was a 2% chance that the cancer could come back in the other breast. I told him that the last four weeks of not knowing were the worst of my life.

"Am I going to die?" I asked. "No, you are not going to die." He replied. "You will need chemotherapy and radiotherapy because of your age to make sure we clear you of the disease, but no, you are not going to die."

He smiled and I knew that I could trust him 110%.

"Does that mean that I will lose my hair?" I asked. "Yes." He replied.

I touched my hair. It was so long that it reached down to the small of my back. My beautiful blonde hair would be gone.

"It's o.k, you can have some of mine." He said. "It's the wrong colour." I replied. "I'm not blonde?" He said smiling. He had dark short hair.

There was a knock at the door, and in came a nurse.

She was introduced as a specialist cancer nurse who would help me through this by answering any questions I had.

The doctor repeated much of our conversation to her.

He then said that I then needed to have a chest x-ray and have some blood taken.

"I'll see you soon." said the doctor as I left. He also gave me a cuddle.

The nurse was fantastic. She took me down to x-ray and booked me in. She was so easy to talk to, like an old friend. We then went and booked me in to have a blood test.

I told her that Steve was outside in the car with Bill and Fred. "Shall I tell him now or after my tests?" I asked her. "It's up to you, but I want you to come and see me after you have had everything done." She said.

I went outside to the car. Bill saw me first, he was bouncing all over the car. "Mum, mum, mum!" He was calling me with a huge smile all over his face. Fred was beaming as well. I took a deep breath. It's good news. I'm not going to die. I kept saying it over and over in my head. As I got to the car, Steve's and my eyes locked. I didn't have to say anything.

"It's going to be alright, babe." He said as he held me close.

"I'm not going to die." I said. "I know." he replied.

I told him that I needed to have some blood taken and an x-ray. "Now?" he asked. "Yes." I replied.

We got the boys out of the car and went back into the hospital. We all went into the x-ray department.

I was called in and asked to put on a gown. I went into the room where they take x-rays. I stood in front of the machine.

"Deep breath. Hold. Thank you." said the nurse.

I went and got dressed and went out to meet Steve. "That was quick." Steve said. "Blood next." I replied. "Upstairs." Off we went.

While we were waiting to have my blood taken I was sitting opposite one of Molly's little friends.

He kept looking at me. I smiled and gave him a wink. They called me in. I sat in a chair with my arm hanging down, the nurse took three tubes of blood, stuck a plaster on me and sent me on my way.

After that we went downstairs to the breast clinic to see my cancer nurse again. We were shown into her office. She won't be long, we were told. Steve and I looked at each other. The tears fell. "It's going to be alright." He said, giving me a big cuddle.

Fred just looked at me with his big blue eyes.

Bill was oblivious to everything and was busy posting leaflets into the drawer of a desk.

It didn't seem real. It was like me looking in on someone else's life.

The nurse came in. She sat down. "Bit of a shock, isn't it." She said. We both nodded. "Have you got any questions?" she asked.

Questions? My mind was a complete blank, it had no questions, not even words or pictures in it, nothing just cotton wool, fuzzy.

We didn't really know what to ask the news was still sinking in. The cancer nurse gave me a card with her telephone number on and said that if or when I had any questions to ring her.

We left the hospital and drove home. Once at home I cried and cried. The tears would not stop.

We put Bill and Fred went upstairs for a nap.

I was not hungry, but instead drank cup after cup of tea.

Steve asked me if I wanted him to phone the 'mums'. I nodded. He went upstairs to make the calls. I went outside in the garden and sat in my greenhouse. It seemed that I just sat there for ages, then from nowhere I felt so angry. Why me. I don't smoke. I don't drink. I haven't done anything really bad. I haven't murdered anyone. Hurt anyone. I don't do drugs, molest children, and beat up old people. Why have I got Cancer?

My Mum had it. My Dad died of it, my Auntie died of it, my Uncle died of it and my Granddad died of it. Isn't that enough for one family?

Haven't we had enough bad luck with people dying before their time? What about people who don't want to live and commit suicide? They could have my cancer and I could have their healthy bodies. People who do drugs, sniff glue, don't care if they live or die, they could have my cancer.

I re-potted my pansies and geraniums. I had to get myself together. The surgeon told me that I wasn't going to die, clear thinking was what was needed. I needed an operation, treatment and recuperation time. Straight forward. Simple.

The surgeon had said they were planning to do the operation at the end of October if everything went to plan. Not long.

I must get the house cleaned, windows washed, garden done. Nothing would be worse that sitting and seeing things that needed to be done and not being able to do them.

Steve came into the garden with another cup of tea.

I could see that he had been crying. I wonder why he won't cry with me?

Jake and Molly came home from school.

"Why were you at the hospital today Mum?" Molly said. I looked at her. "How did you know I was there?" I asked. "My friend saw you and he said that you were crying." She said. "Oh" I replied.

I didn't know what to say, so I asked her how her football training had gone, and she chatted happily about what had happened.

Later when Jake and Molly had gone out to play, I rang the 'mums'. I said that I was fine. No, they didn't have to visit. Yes, we would carry on life as normal and no, we were not going to tell Jake and Molly. Life just carried on.

Jake and Molly went to their Friday night club and Steve went up the pub.

I stayed in on my own, just as normal.

September 25th

An advert in the paper caught my eye. It was for a Spiritual Healer. It took place every Saturday morning in a hall just up the road from us. I organised the children and went to see what it was all about.

When I got to the hall it was taking place in one of the rooms upstairs.

As I went up the stairs I could hear harp music. It made me think of waterfalls. I stood in the doorway, I felt nervous about going in. There were about eight old ladies sitting round a large table drinking tea. From around the corner appeared a man. "Are you waiting for someone?" He asked. "No, I saw your advert in the paper and thought I would come and see you." I replied. "Oh, come on in then." He said smiling.

He led me into the room. He sat me next to a lady. She introduced herself. "Welcome to the group, would you like a cup of tea." She asked.

"Yes please." I replied. I looked around, I wondered to myself what I was doing there, were they weirdo's spouting mumbo jumbo?

The man who had introduced me into the group said that they were about to begin. Everybody bowed their heads. He said a prayer. Tears welled up in my eyes and began to fall. I felt a tissue placed in my hand and I opened my eyes. In front of me there was a lady looking at me. She had the kindest eyes and face I had ever seen. I felt that I could share anything with her. She held my hands. "I've got cancer." I said. It was the first time I had said it out aloud. "Oh, my sweet." said the lady. She gave me a cuddle.

"I am a healer. Would you like to be healed?"

I just looked at her. "Come on." She said.

She led me over to where two chairs were facing each other and I sat down. She placed her hands on my knees and looked into my eyes.

"Where have they found it?" She said. "In the breast." I replied. "When did you find out?" She asked. "Yesterday morning." I said.

She squeezed my knees. She explained what she was going to do.

"I'll start at the top of your head and work down your body, placing my hands on you. While I am healing, think of somewhere you are totally relaxed and secure. Somewhere you feel safe."

I closed my eyes and the image of my dads face came into my head. Not his whole face, just his nose, mouth and chin. 'Oh Dad,' my mind shouted, 'why aren't you here. I need you so much!' The tears came again.

The lady started healing She started by placing her hands on the top of my head, then round the sides, over my ears, over my eyes, on my jaw, round my neck, on my shoulders. As she moved down my body the tears seemed to fade away. She carried on until she had made her way down to my feet. She placed her hands on my breast again. A warm feeling came into it. She held my hands. "Open your eyes." she asked. I opened my eyes and we smiled at each other. I put my hand on my breast. "It went all warm when you placed your hands here." I said. "That's the healing." She replied. "We don't tell you what to expect, we wait for you to tell us. The warmth is the healing working. Will you come and see us next week?" She asked. "Yes." I replied. "Every night I will pray for your healing," she said "and every day place your hand on your breast and ask the Divine Spirit to heal you."

I said thank you and felt soothed as if I had been taken away the harshness of the reality. It made me feel that I was not facing this on my own.

I walked home feeling strangely calm. The tears seemed to have gone deeper inside rather than being so near to the surface that they threaten nearly every time I blinked.

Lucy came down to stay in the afternoon.

Steve told her the news when she went upstairs to put her bag in her bedroom. She was shocked and asked him if I was going to die. He explained what had happened and what was going to be done. She went very quiet.

September 26th

John came round as usual for his lunch. Steve told him after lunch and his reaction was to get very angry. "Why?" Was all he kept saying He started to cry. I went in and gave him a cuddle."You realize that when my hair goes, yours has to go as well because you can't have longer hair than me." "It's not funny." He said, "It's not fair, just not fair."

The reaction the people have when they are told that you have cancer is strange to see. I remember when my Dad told me. Your first feeling is disbelief, you can't believe that someone so close to you has cancer, then you feel a terrible rage, cancer happens to people that you don't known not someone you love, the last feeling is one of panic when you realize that this person in front of you could die and you are totally powerless to prevent it. People avoid eye contact with you after that, maybe it is because the eyes are the doorway to the soul and they don't want to see your pain.

Body language can lie and deceive, but the eyes always tell the truth. The truth always hurts and people don't like to be hurt.

September 29th

I'd been thinking since I found the lump that if it was cancer that I would have my haircut before the treatment started. That way it would be easier on the children rather than me going from having long hair to nothing.

The next morning before the children went to school I went over the road to see a lady who is a hairdresser. I asked her if she would cut my hair. She suggested that I had it cut in a bob first and then once I had got used to it have it cut again. I said that I wanted it all cut off at the same time. She asked why. I took a deep breath and told her the reason. She said of course she would do it and she said that she would come over and cut it later that morning.

When I got back home I asked Molly to take a photograph of me with my hair down. She asked why and I told her it was a surprise.

After Jake and Molly went to school the lady came over, I had put my hair up in a ponytail and plaited it. She took hold of it and cut it off. I put it on the counter and looked at it. It looked yucky!

It looked like part of my body on the side that was not attached to me. I didn't know whether to keep it or not, so wrapped it in a bag and put it in the draw. Maybe I could sell it to a wig maker?

She began cutting my hair and we chatted away.

"Finished." she said. I got up and looked in the mirror. "That's brilliant!" I said. "Thank you ever so much."

My hair was cut close to the sides and a couple of inches longer on the top. She would not take any money for doing it, so later in the day I went and bought her some flowers.

Jake wasn't impressed when he saw me. He said that I didn't look like his mum any more. "You'll get used to it, Jake." I told him. "Soon it will be normal and the photos of me with long hair will look weird."

Molly just laughed. "I don't know what you're laughing about!" I told her. "Yours is next." That made her go quiet. When Steve came home from work he said it looked lovely but that I should wear earrings, as from the back I looked like a bloke!

It felt weird not having hair. Especially when I put a jumper on, or lay down, but it is much easier and quicker to look after….except, that I look like 'Stan Laurel' in the morning with no effort at all!

September 30ᵗʰ

My first appointment with my surgeon. He was very handsome and looked dashing in his suit. He would look at home in Harley Street.

He had an air of complete confidence about him that almost made you want to call him 'sir'.

When I met him I knew that I was in very capable hands.

He examined me and then sat me down. He explained again the different options. I could have the lump removed, but, if they did not remove it all I would then need a second operation. I could have the whole breast removed which would include the nipple, or I could have the breast removed and have it reconstructed using muscle from my back. I had already decided that I wanted both breasts removed. I told him what I had decided. "If you are quite sure, then we have to make sure the disease has not spread, as we would be taking away healthy tissue and if it has gone anywhere else those places would take priority, we will do a bone scan and a liver scan, you have already had a chest scan. If the other scans come back clear we will do a double mastectomy for you." He said. "If it is anywhere else can you treat it?" I asked. He looked at me. "No, we cannot. We can only manage it, not cure it." "Well lets hope that it's no where else then." I replied.

There was a different breast cancer nurse there that time and after I had left the surgeon she took me into another room to 'discuss' how I was dealing with my situation. I sat down with her. "That was so cruel." I started. "I had been told that I had cancer, but it had been caught and that I wasn't going to die. Now I'm being told if it is somewhere else, then, I'm sorry Mrs Bond there is nothing we can do for you!

Everything so far I have been able to cope with, but, what he has just said puts me right back to the beginning again.

It's so unfair. I now have to go back to my family and pretend that everything is normal, when I just want to disappear, but, I can't and tomorrow I have to smile and laugh with Fred because it's his birthday. All I want to do is go somewhere and scream. How do I do that when I don't know whether this thing inside me is slowly making me die?" She sat there and nodded. She said all the right things, gave me tissues and promised to ring in the morning when she had sorted out the scans.

October

October 1ˢᵗ
HAPPY 1ˢᵗ BIRTHDAY FRED!

As promised the nurse rang me. She asked how I was. "Still smiling." I replied."Good." She said. "Now I have booked your bone scans for Monday. You will need to come in at 11am for an injection and then come back for the scan at 3pm. The liver scan has been booked for today at 2pm. Can you make that?" I told her that I could. "Good," she said again. "and then on Friday you will see the surgeon for the results."

I thanked her ever so much and carried on with the day.

Mum and Dad came over for Fred's birthday.

At 2pm Dad took me to the hospital for the scan. We didn't wait long before I was called in. I laid down on the couch. The lady asked me to pull up my top, they checked my name and address and left me, saying the radiologist would be in, in a minute.

I laid there and looked at the ceiling, making all kinds of deals with God if he made the scan come out all right. The radiologist came in, she was ever so nice. We had a chat while she was doing checks on me. I told her it was Freds Birthday today and she asked how many children I had. .

She must have felt my heart going balmy because she told me to take some deep breaths. "Is the scan all right?" I asked. I couldn't breath as I waited for the answer. She gave me a big smile.

"It looks fine, totally normal." "Ohhhhh!" I breathed out. My heart flew up and down and did somersaults. The relief went from my head to my toes and back again. "That's the best birthday present I could give Fred." I blubbed.

Talk about being a drama queen!.

She showed me on the screen all the bits of the liver. "The large node is on the right side just under the ribs. The smaller node is on the left with the gall bladder in the middle. Sparkly bits are normal, the little black holes are ducts." she explained.

I went back into the waiting room. The smile on my face was so huge, dad didn't need to ask if everything was all right. We went home very happy.

When we got home mum met us at the door. "You can't come in," She said anxiously.

"Why not?" I said. "Have you got a surprise for me?" Mum hesitated.

"Not exactly, I turned on the tap in the kitchen to do the washing up," she began, "and then I heard Bill upstairs and when I got back downstairs there was water everywhere!"

Fred had been in his walker and had been running through it. The counters were dripping and it had gone in the drawers and in the cupboards and filled up the saucepans.

"Good job we were only half an hour." I said, getting some newspaper to put on the floor. We told Mum the good news, we had a big cuddle. I went upstairs to ring Steve, and then my Mum and John.

We all had a nice cup of tea. Jake and Molly came home from school. We lit the candles on Freds birthday cake. Fred blew out the candles with the help of Bill and opened his presents with the help of Jake and Molly.

Mum and Dad said that it would be fine to have the boys on Monday.

This was because the bone scan involved having radiation injected into your body and you are not allowed to cuddle small children for twenty-four hours.

I got their things together and they went home with Mum and Dad.

Jake and Molly were going away also, so it was not long before I found myself......childless!

October 4th

Steve came to the hospital and with me for the injection at 11:30am. We had to go to the Nuclear Medicine Department. It was really strange. It was like walking into a science-fiction film. There were lots of radiation signs around and notices warning of contamination. They asked me my name and address and date of birth. I had to sign a form to say that I wasn't pregnant. They then injected me with radiation. I was told I could eat and drink normally, they also said that they had a cancellation so I could come back earlier than expected. They would see me at 2pm.

We went home. Steve cut the grass and I went shopping.

When we got back to the hospital we had to wait quite a while because there was someone in there. It was my turn to go in. I went into a room there was a bed in the middle. At the end of the bed there were two scanners, one above and one underneath. I was told to lie down and turn my head to the left. They lowered the scanning machine over my head. "Don't worry." said the nurse. "It won't squash you. It has sensors that make it stop." It stopped just resting on my face…It was not a very nice experience! I was told that the scan would take seventeen minutes and forty three seconds. The nurse brought down a screen with 17:43 on it so that I could see when it would be finished.

The scanner moved very slowly all the way down to my toes. When it had finished I was told that my left knee needed to be done again. They bent it and scanned it again. They apologised and said that they could not get a clear picture and had booked me into have an x-ray taken of it and would I make my way down to the x-ray department as they were expecting me. One of the nurses walked with me and asked if she could be rung when I had finished. The x-ray department was really busy and we had to wait ages to be seen, eventually I was. They took two x-rays and I was told to wait outside. They told me they were not clear enough and I had to have more taken. They took some more and I was told to wait outside again. While I was waiting two nurses from the radiology department came and found me. They apologised for the waiting around and explained that several of them had been looking at my x-rays and had decided that what they could see on my knee was nothing to do with cancer and that they thought that is was the early stages of arthritis.

I went home feeling flat. I had been really happy after my liver scan and this result was just as good, but I just felt nothing. I got home and I didn't want to speak to any one. I just curled myself up on the sofa. I was so fed up with the not knowing. I had to wait until Friday.

October 5th

HAPPY BIRTHDAY MUM!

Today I got a letter from the hospital with the date for my operation. It says that I would be going in on the 18th October at 2pm. That means that all the tests had come through clear! The surgeon had said that they would only operate if it was nowhere else. I cried. But this time it was with relief. Soon this nightmare would be over.

I rang the breast care nurse that had arranged the scans for me and told her about the letter. "That means that all the scans are clear, doesn't it?" I said."Not necessary," she said, "all it means is that your operation has been booked in…,hang on, let me check and see if your results are in."

I hung on the phone. "You know about the liver scan don't you?" She asked. "Yes." I replied.

"Your chest x-ray has also come through clear. Your heart is normal, not enlarged and there are no nodes in the lungs. The only results we haven't got are the bone scans that you had done yesterday. How did it go?" She asked. I explained what had happened. She said that she would let me know the minute they had my results of my bone scan. I then rang everyone with the good news about the chest x-ray.

October 8th

This is the day I find out what is what. My appointment is at 10am. Steve and I got there on time and we were seen straight away. The surgeon, my breast care nurse and another nurse were all in the room. I didn't know whether that was a good or bad sign. The surgeon shook our hands. I asked about the results. "All the results are fine, normal." said the surgeon. I breathed out a huge sigh of relief and a few drippy tears. In my head I had an image of a little man jumping up and down shouting 'You're not going to die, you're not going to die!'

"You have caused us a bit of head scratching, though." The surgeon said. "Regarding your knee. At the moment your bone scan and x-rays are at Oxford as we don't know what it is, but we know that it isn't cancer because…..."

He put a picture of the scan up on the computer for us all to see. "If it was cancer, the shape of the bone would look as if it had been eaten away and yours is the shape it should be, but, it looks as if you have some fuzzy, cotton-wool stuff in your bone that we can't identify."

That was all right then …I think?

We then chatted about the operation, because I was having a double mastectomy they would not be able to use muscle from my back as there would not be enough to do both breasts, so, they were going to remove the breast tissue and the nipples as they are made of the same cells as the inside of the breast, not the skin on the outside. Place implants underneath my pectoral muscles to stretch them, then at a later date they would be able to give me some proper ones, called 'jellybeans' and nipple reconstruction once everything was over. They would use skin from 'down below' and tattoo it, so it looked more like a proper nipple. He also said that the operation would be going ahead on the 19th as planned.

We all shook hands and with big smiles on our faces, we went home.

I was so happy, on the way home a great wave of relief swept over me and I seemed to melt into the chair. Now we knew what we were up against and there were no hidden surprises waiting to jump out on us.

October 13th

Today I had an appointment with the sister on the ward where I would have the operation. I went up to the ward and was met by her.

My heart missed a beat because this was the ward that I came to New Years Day 2002 and had a scan. I had lost the baby I was carrying.

We sat down and she showed me pictures of the operation and what I would look like after.

She said that I would be on oxygen for one day, morphine for three days, have three or four drains coming out of me by my breasts and armpits and be in for at least a week.

She also said that because I was having the lymph nodes removed from my right armpit, I would always have to be careful. If I got a cut or a scratch on that arm I would have to wash it really well and put on some germoline to make sure that I didn't get an infection, because, if I did my arm would swell up and they might not be able to make the swelling go away.

This is when the reality hit me. Up until now it had been like this was happening to someone else, as if it was surreal, a nasty dream, that I would wake up from and think, thank goodness that wasn't real and carry on with my life. Now it was happening to me.

I started crying. The sister said that it was a normal reaction and all the ladies going through this operation felt the same. I asked if it was a common operation and she replied that it was happening more and more.

I was then weighed and had some blood taken. She asked me lots of questions like: Had I had any operation before? Was I allergic to anything? and other questions. I had to go to some different departments and have some blood taken and an E.C.G, so they knew what my normal heart rhythm was.

I went home very apprehensive. I knew that she was telling me the worst scenario possible, but, the difference between the surgeon saying I would be a bit ' uncomfortable' and how the sister explained it, were worlds apart.

October 15ᵗʰ

Went to a friends Wedding for the weekend.

We stayed in a lovely country hotel. The weather was good and they had the ceremony and the reception there.

In the evening they had a disco but I went to bed early as I felt the whole situation was unreal, here I was enjoying their celebration knowing that I had cancer and that in two days time I would be having both my breasts removed to stop the disease from killing me! How surreal is that? I looked around and thought if only we knew what other people were thinking and feeling the burden some of them are carrying while smiling, you would never know. Nobody would ever guess what was going round my head, to them I am just another person enjoying the wedding of a friend with my family.

Maybe it is better that we don't know what is going on in peoples heads. Anyway we had a wonderful time, she looked beautiful and he was very handsome, the children behaved themselves. The sun shined, just as it should do.

Chapter 2.

October 18th

Rang the ward at 1pm, to be told that there wasn't a bed available for me and to ring back again at 4pm.

I rang again at 4pm, and was told that they had a bed for me and that it was in a side room. They said that I could go in at any-time.

I had picked my Mum up from the coach station in the morning.

After we all had our tea, Jake and Molly went out to play. I bathed the boys, said goodbye to my Mum, then Steve took me to the hospital.

Once in the ward I was shown to my room and told to make myself comfortable. I put my case down and sat on the bed. This is it, I thought. It's really happening.

A large smiley nurse came in and introduced herself. She read my details out to make sure that I was me, then she put an identity bracelet with my name and hospital number on my wrist. She also gave me some white stockings to wear.

She said that I had to wear them all the time I was in hospital, to minimize the risk of blood clots as I would be spending a lot of time in bed.

She took my blood pressure, oxygen levels, and then my temperature.

Steve had his oxygen levels taken as well, his was 98% and mine was 100%. After that she left us alone.

The drinks lady came round and we had a cup of tea, made the television work and then Steve went home. "I'll be back in the morning, sweet'eart." He said, giving me a kiss and cuddle.

I got undressed, washed and settled myself into bed. It was so quiet there after the noise of home it took ages for me to go to sleep.

Weighed 8st 5lbs.

October 19th

I was awake early and had a nice shower. The nurse came in and took my blood pressure and temperature. Then the surgeon came in. He asked if I understood what would be happening today. I said that I did. He asked me to remove my top. He then got out a marker pen.

"Would you mind if I draw on you?" He said. "Don't worry its not where I'm going to cut, it's just the shape of the breasts because it changes once you lay down."

We had a bit of a chat and another man came in, who introduced himself and said he would be assisting the surgeon during the operation.

"See you in a bit." he said, and then left.

The door knocked again and in came another man who introduced himself as the anaesthetist.

He told me he would be looking after me until I went into the recovery room. He asked me lots of questions about my breathing, heart, liver and problems with my stomach, like indigestion.

He also told me that his sister had had the same operation as me about five years ago, and that she was perfectly fine now. As he left, Steve came in.

We had a kiss and cuddle. We hadn't finished before there was another knock at the door and a trolley was wheeled in.

"We are ready to take you down." said a lady porter.

It felt like I was being rushed. Everything seemed to be happening at once.

They put me on the trolley and took me down the corridor into a lift and then down another corridor. The lady porter and Steve were discussing the hospital, soon we got to a double set of doors.

"This is where you say goodbye." she said to Steve. "You can't come any further." I looked at him and tears welled up in my eyes. We said our goodbyes with a cuddle. "You'll be fine." Steve said, "I'll be right out side waiting for you."

As they wheeled me through the doors we both said, "I love you."(Yucky slushy bit!)

I was pushed into another room where I met a lady who worked with the anaesthetist. She asked me my name and date of birth. They transferred me onto another thin trolley and I was taken into another room. The anaesthetist who I had met in my room was in there. "Hello again." he said.

They put a cannula in my left hand and they had to ask the surgeon where he wanted them to put the other cannula and he told them to put it in my right foot, that was for the morphine (P.C.A.). We were all talking about our children, when the anaesthetist put some liquid into the cannula in my left hand and............

I remember waking up confused. I was told that it was all over. All over? It can't be? I heard different people calling my name. I saw faces that I didn't recognise. I couldn't move. It felt like there was a huge weight on my chest. Then the pain hit me, from under my armpits and across my chest. I remember saying that it hurt. Someone put something in my hand, "Press the button." I was told and I did. The pain went away. I felt them moving me, along the corridor, over the bumps. The pain came again."Press the button." I was told again. We stopped moving. I heard Steve's voice. He smoothed my hair. He removed the oxygen mask and gave me a kiss. The pain came again."Press the button." I was told. Where was the button? I couldn't move. Voices were talking, I thought I heard my mum. Nothing now, just sleep. It was night-time. I had a blood pressure sleeve on my leg. It kept working, squeezing my leg, bleeping, relaxing. I went back to sleep. It kept doing that all through the night.

Where I had had the lymph nodes taken from my right arm arm I can not longer use that arm for things like blood tests and blood pressure readings, as any trauma to the arm would make the lymph system work and because it has been removed it would send some from somewhere else causing a build up of fluid, which, would make my arm swell like a balloon and it wouldn't do me much good.

I had a drain running from the side of each breast into containers so they could measure how much blood and other stuff was emptying into them. I had a catheter, a cannula in my left hand and a P.C.A cannula in the top of my right foot which was administering morphine when I pressed a button.

October 20th

"Morning!" I was greeted by a very happy nurse. "Today we are going to get you up, washed and sitting in a chair for an hour." she said. "I don't think so," I replied. " I'm going back to sleep."

They got the controls for my bed and moved the back of it, so that they had me sitting up. The pain in my chest was horrible. I couldn't move properly. I couldn't move my arms, the pain was so awful. They told me to use the P.C.A as it would go away in a few minutes. I didn't want to use the button. The auxiliary nurse came in to give me a wash. I didn't want to move because I knew that it was going to hurt. My eyes couldn't focus on anything, they kept on going blurry. The nurse helped me move my legs round so that I was sitting up on the side of the bed. That was enough."I'm going to be sick,!" I announced.

They told me to take a deep breath. I tried, but it hurt and my chest was so tight that I couldn't do it very well. I coughed and heaved, but I didn't have the strength in my chest to do anything. I made a few pathetic attempts, during this there was a knock at the door. A nurse said that my Mum was on the phone, asking how I was. "Oh, I can see." she said backing out of the door.

The auxiliary nurse opened a window and after a while I began to feel better. I was still sitting up. I felt extremely sleepy. I didn't want a cup of tea or any breakfast. Just sleep. At lunchtime I had a roll and a few mouthfuls of soup. I thought that it would make me feel better as I was still feeling sick.

The lady came in from the blood clinic and took some blood from my left foot, she stuck the needle in near my little toe........That was so painful! Then the nurse came and took the P.C.A. cannula out of my right foot.

Steve came in to see me in the afternoon and was surprised to see me sitting up.

He gave me a kiss and kept looking at me.

"You look weird." He said. "Your hair is flat against your head and sticking up at the back and your face is all puffy." He looked at me closer.

"It looks like you haven't got any eyebrows, but you have." I laughed. "You know how to make me feel better don't you." He laughed too. "I didn't expect to see you sitting up after how you were yesterday." he exclaimed.

I kept falling asleep while he was there. "I've got to go in a bit," he said. "Mum and Dad are coming over and they want to pop in and see that you are alright." He gave me a kiss and left.

I must have fallen asleep again as I was woken up by them bringing in my supper, I had just started eating my soup and roll, when Steve came in again. "Mum and Dad are outside, they want to see you, only for a minute, just to put their minds at rest." He looked at me for an answer. "Alright." I said. Mum and Dad came in. I gave them a big smile. "Oh, my babe." Mum said giving me a hug as best she could. Dad stood at the end of my bed and looked at me. "Well it looks like no more cakes for a couple of weeks then?" He said "Now that we have seen that you are alright we will leave you." They both gave me a kiss and left. Steve said that he was going home for his tea and also left. I was alone again, I fell asleep.

Steve came back in the evening and stayed until he was asked to leave. After he had left I couldn't sleep. The cannula in my left hand had become red and sore so the nurse took it out. I looked at the clock it said 12:45am.

October 21st

I kept waking up and got up about 5:30am. I made the bed sit up and I shuffled my bottom up the bed until I was sitting up. My chest still felt really tight and sore and every time I moved I felt the blood and stuff go through the drains under my arms, especially the left one. It felt really warm and weird. The pain in my chest wasn't as bad as yesterday. Taking a deep breath, I moved my legs around until I was sitting up at the side of the bed. I lent over the side and picked up my left drain, then I lent over and picked up my right drain and catheter. Taking a deep breath I stood up. I waited a moment, I didn't feel dizzy or sick.

I slowly walked to the bathroom. Once inside the bathroom I moved the stool over and sat down. I took some deep breath, made it.

I cleaned my teeth that felt better. I decided to have a go at washing. First I did my face and then gently took off my nightie and washed my tummy and under my arms. The left one was o.k, a bit sore, but the right armpit was completely numb. I also had what felt like 'bolts', one on either side, they were in line with the bottom of my breasts. I washed my underneath and finally I washed my hair. My arms were a bit sore at the beginning, but as I washed, my arms felt easier.

All done I got myself changed into a clean set of pyjamas and walked back to my bed. I got back into bed and fell asleep.

The nurse came in and took my blood pressure and temperature, she also gave me an injection in my left thigh, which, she said stopped blood clots.

A doctor came round and checked my dressings and the amount of fluid that had gone into the drains. "You are doing fine." he said. "The right drain can come out today. Very good. Any problems?" "No." I replied. He promised that it would not hurt having the drain taken out. He said, that it would feel like a slight scratch. "Not that I've ever had one removed," he hastened to add! He smiled and left the room. I had my breakfast and settled down for the day. The physiotherapist came round to see me. She gave me a leaflet on exercises that I should be doing in the morning and the evening.

She asked me to raise my arms, in the front, at my sides, and the back. I did them all. "Well done!" she said.

She was surprised that I could do all the exercises so easily. She stayed and had a chat, then she said that she had to go, but would be back tomorrow.

Lunch came and then a nurse came in and said that she was going to take out the drain. She was just about to start when Steve came in. She laid the bed flat and asked me to slip my top over my arm so she could reach it. She talked me through what she was doing. First she cut the stitch, and then she took off the dressing. She asked me to take some deep breaths and on the third one, she pulled the drainage tube. I was surprised that it didn't hurt because it had been so tender. But it just felt like a release. Later another nurse came in and took out the catheter.

The lady that comes round with a cup of tea after every meal and again in the afternoons keeps making me laugh. Every time she pops her head round the door I always seem to have my ankles crossed and she keeps telling me off.

It's not too bad here everyone is always coming in for chats, I even had a visit from the lady porter that took me down for my operation!

October 22ⁿᵈ

I woke up later than yesterday, and had a much better nights sleep. I went to the bathroom, I felt that I needed the toilet but I seem to be a bit bunged up, it took ages. I had a full wash, which was much easier then yesterday. I was just going to start my breakfast when my surgeon came in.

He asked how I was and said that the surgeon with the bow-tie asked him to send me his regards. He checked my drain and told me that it could come out today. He then looked at my chest and was pleased at what he saw.

I was surprised that he was because when I looked down all I could see was that I was completely black and blue from my collar bone down to my hips!

"How can you be pleased?" I asked him. "Look at the state of me! It looks like you have jumped up and down all over me!"

He gave me a knowing look and a small smile.

"You are doing really well, in fact you can go home tomorrow." I just looked at him.

"Don't you want to go home?" He asked.

"Steve said for me to go home on Sunday." I replied.

How stupid did that sound? It was bad enough that he made you feel that you should have at least brushed your hair before he came in, let alone saying something as daft as that. Where is that huge hole that you just want to jump in to when you need it?

Although I couldn't wait to go home, being told I could, made me nervous of the real world. In here I was being looked after, I didn't have to worry about anything, outside I had to return to being Mum and I didn't know if I was ready to have all the responsibility back on my shoulders again.

I know that my mum is there but anything that needed a decision on, she would ask me.

I rang the children and had a nice chat with Molly and Bill, Jake was out playing.

The nurse came round and gave me my medicines and an injection in my leg. She said that she would be round later to take out the drain.

I don't seem to be able to concentrate on anything, the days are just blurring into each other.

I picked my nose today and found a bogey. I can't remember the last time that I had had one of those, but it was ages ago. I wonder if the cancer stops you having them? Does that mean that all the cancer has gone then if the bogeys have returned?

The nurse came in to take out the drain, she was ever so nice. She comes from Australia. She was chatting as she got everything ready and she was just about to start when Steve came in. He had come in because he had no money, it was in the purse in my bag. "Oh good." I said, "now that you are here you can hold my hand while the nurse takes out the drain." I told him what the surgeon had said about me going home early and he just smiled.

"Right," said the nurse. "On the third deep breath I will remove the drain." I squeezed Steve's hand and breathed deeply. "Bananas." Steve whispered in my ear. I smiled. "All done." said the nurse.

"That didn't hurt at all." I said. "No, it shouldn't," she replied. "It should just feel a bit weird."

This time it had felt like a big spot being squeezed and the relief was lovely.

Steve left, then the nurse left after she had dressed the hole where the drain had come from.

I had my lunch, then went to the toilet again as I am having trouble going.

I have grown a large lump on my right hand side like a huge 'love-handle'. Looking down my body resembles part of the elephant man. It is really tender and sore. I look most attractive, being disfigured and black and blue, with a slight hint of yellow!

I was in the bathroom when Mum and Dad turned up. They were early as visiting doesn't start until 2 o'clock. They stayed for about an hour telling me all the gossip and things that were going on. They asked how long I would be in for and said they would come and see me on Monday either here or at home.

When they left, I felt tired and kept getting waves of feeling sick.

I was feeling a bit sorry for myself. I had started to cry this morning when the nurse came in. I don't know why but I keep on crying, maybe it's normal as I did have a long operation, only two days ago.

There was a knock at the door. My Mum bounced in. "Ta-da!" She said all smiley. "Hello, Mum." I said. We had a big cuddle. "Don't you look well?" she said, as she flopped in the chair. We talked about the pleasures of having four children and Steve at home.

Time went really quickly and soon she said she had to go and get the tea on the table by 5 o'clock, 'routine, routine', as Steve would say!

We had another cuddle and she went home. I stood at the window and waved to her as she went to the car. As I lifted my left arm to wave, I felt a 'whoosh' sensation in my armpit. The same sensation that I had felt when the drains were in and the fluid was coming out. I went into the bathroom and lifted my top. I looked in the mirror.

It was the first time that I had seen my chest from this angle as I had seen it when looking down at it. Looking at it through my top it didn't look any different than it had before the operation. But without my top on, it was a shock. The shape of them wasn't that different, but it was the colour. Under my boobs it was a deep red and purple colour, it shocked me because it was much worse on the left side where I had had the 'woosh' feeling. I covered myself up and went back to bed. I knew that I should tell someone but I didn't want them to say that I needed something else done to me.

As I was thinking this, the nurse that had taken out my drain earlier came in. I decided to show her as, what I had was quite serious in the first place. I told her what had happened and showed her my chest. She took a good look and felt it all over. She told me that it all looked fine, but to put my mind at rest she would get someone else to come in and double-check it for me.

The Sister came and agreed with her it was normal. I showed them my new 'love-handle' and asked them if that was normal as well. They asked me if I had had a bowel movement. I said that I had had a couple of small ones. "You're bunged up." they said. "You need to have a good poo. When was the last time you went properly?"

"Tuesday morning." I replied. It was now Friday afternoon. "No wonder you are feeling uncomfortable." They said. We had a laugh about it and they threatened me with suppositories.

"No, you're all right." I said. They then suggested lactolose. I accepted the offer of the 'old ladies medicine'. They smiled and left the room.

Steve came in. "Busy day?" I asked. He chuckled. He gave me some cards that the children had made for me, there was one from Molly and all the children in her class and some from her and Bill, Fred and Jake. Steve also gave me a postcard photo thing that he had done at the shops. It has a photo of him on it and the words 'I love you.' Talk about pull at the heart-strings!

It was lovely and extra special as it is not the sort of soppy thing he does. I asked for a cuddle. It felt wonderful. He smoothed my back and I began to feel loved again. It was a fantastic feeling. I showed him my 'love-handle' and said that I needed some exercise to get things moving, but he wouldn't come for a walk down the corridor, so I walked up and down my room.

I felt like a prisoner, I was ready to go home, just like the surgeon had said. Steve stayed for a while, but, it was Friday night and that's his night to be out. We had another cuddle and he went home. I watched him go to the car from the window. I felt a bit sad.

October 23rd

I woke early this morning at 4 o'clock. I felt terrible; I can't explain how I felt it was just yucky. I got up and went to the bathroom and tried to go to the toilet again without any luck.

I decided to go out and see one of the nurses on duty and ask for some suppositories. She asked if I wanted her to do them. "No thank you," I said. "I'll do it myself." So, armed with rubber gloves I went back to my room and did the yucky job .... with my eyes closed!.

I got into bed and watched television waiting for them to do their work.

Result! I got back into bed, feeling slightly better.

I must have fallen asleep again because I was woken by the nurse who had come to give me my injection. She asked if I had been successful. I told her that I had. After the nurse had gone I went back into the bathroom. They were working wonders. I had a nice hot wash, washed my hair and put on some clean pyjamas.

When I came out there was another nurse in my room waiting to take my blood pressure and   temperature.

I kept looking at her because she looked really familiar. Then it came to me. She belonged to the dance class Steve and I went to on a Sunday evening. It took her longer to recognise me because the last time she had seen me I had long hair.

We chatted about this and that then she said that she had to go and do the rest of the ward.

I rang home and spoke to Molly and Bill, Jake was out playing again. I told them that I was coming home tomorrow. Molly was pleased with the news and Bill told me that he was going up to the shops to get a paper!

I did my arm exercises and some jogging up and down my room, how sad. Jogging!

My right shoulder is playing up today.

I had my lunch and some more lactalose and rested on my bed watching television. A nurse came in and took my blood pressure and temperature and a doctor came in and took some blood from me. Steve came in to see me and told me that they were having fish and chips for tea.

October 24ᵗʰ

Woke up at 3 o'clock this morning. I can't seem to sleep properly, so I watched a bit of television.

The nurse came in at 7 o'clock and gave me my injection. I had a cup of tea and then got washed. Today my 'bowel habits' are back to normal, thank goodness. I put my trousers and a t-shirt because I'm going home!

I was packing when the nurse came in, she said that my blood count was low, 8:7 and that they would have to re-do it again because if it hadn't picked up there was a chance I would need a transfusion. She said it was done through a cannula in my left hand and that I would need two or three bags, which take three to four hours each. I cross my fingers that it would come back better.

I rang Steve and told him what the nurse had said. Frustration made me cry telling him.

Every morning it has been the same, a few tears, so silly. The worst bit is over …..I hope.

I did my exercises. They weren't as easy as yesterday. I had a go at doing some yoga probably didn't do it right but it made me feel a bit better. I must get more supple….. It does hurt. I will be all right when I get home.

The nurse came in and said that my blood count was now 8:8 and that I needed a transfusion. I rang Steve, I'm so upset. The tears came thick and fast. I wanted to go home, not stay another day. I had my lunch. My Mum and John came to see me. At 4:30pm the doctor came round he said that although my count was low, (normally it would be between 12 and 14) they only do transfusions if the count is under 8 and in his opinion I was o.k to go home. He said that he would give me a letter for the district nurse, she would change my dressings in a couple of days. I thanked him.

The nurse came back with some iron tablets for me to take. She also changed my dressings where the drain had been. They had been slightly leaking so she thought that it was best. She said that I needed to come back in the morning as they didn't have enough iron tablets there for the amount that had been prescribed by the doctor.

I looked at John. "Can you take me home please?" I asked. He smiled. We all walked down to the car park. I was surprised how weak my arms were. I could not pull or push the doors, mum had to open them for me.

It was raining outside. John ran ahead and got the car while me and mum waited under the covered doorway.

I took loads of deep breaths. It was the most wonderful feeling, fresh air and rain. It made me feel so alive. I tilted my head up to the sky and let the rain fall on me. I felt so lucky to be outside.

I arrived home to loads of cuddles and kisses.

HOME SWEET HOME!

Weight 8st 10lbs.

Chapter 3

October 25th

Woke up at 7 o'clock. It's lovely to be at home, but it hurts so much.

I didn't realize how much the bed in hospital had helped me. It made me cry sitting up. My muscles were so stiff and sore. It hurt just moving. I noticed that there was a swelling under my right armpit. I showed Mum and she said that we would mention it when we went to the hospital later.

Mum made me some tea and toast. I did my exercises and took some painkillers.

I got up and went downstairs to help Mum with Bill and Fred. I changed Bills nappy and gave Fred his breakfast. I ran the bath and got in breathing a huge sigh of relief. Home. My Home.

I went with Mum to the hospital to get the rest of my iron tablets. I saw the sister and she asked me how I was. I told her that it was hurting more than it did when I was in hospital. I showed her where it had become swollen under my right armpit. She rang the breast nurse and she came to have a look. She said that she thought that it was fine but she wanted the doctor to come and have a look.

The doctor came and had a look. He said that it was because there was more scar tissue on that side. It was where they had removed the lymph nodes and it would settle down. He was surprised at the amount of bruising that I had. He prescribed some antibiotics just to be on

29

the safe side. So I came home with iron tablets, paracetamol and anti-inflammatory tablets, later I would pick up the antibiotics.

Mum and Dad came over as arranged to see me. They brought some flowers. They made me cry. Auntie Sylvia rang and asked how I was.

Weighed 8st 8lbs.

October 26th

Steve went back to work today. I had my breakfast early and took all the tablets I was supposed to. I had a snooze and felt fantastic. I think it is the anti-inflammatory tablets that make all the difference.

Mum took Bill shopping so I thought that I would do the ironing. I took the ironing board off its hook. It didn't hurt, so I carried on. I ended up ironing the whole basket of clothes. Had a sleep in the afternoon.

Lucy had spent the weekend with us, so in the evening Steve and I drove her home. I had felt 'not right' all afternoon and thought that the drive might make me feel a bit better, or, at least take my mind of it.

That night I had an awful tummy ache. It felt like really bad period pains. I had a hot water bottle as I couldn't take any more painkillers. Later that night I had terrible diarrhoea and after four times my stomach felt better and so did I.

October 27th

Woke up feeling better and found it easier to move than I had yesterday. My stomach is a bit sore. Went to the toilet, that's gone back to normal. Had all my tablets, made Mum some breakfast.

Got a letter in the post for my next consultation, next Wednesday at 3:30pm.

The district nurse came round to change the dressing. She said that the left drain hole was looking a bit 'mankey'. Well that's what she called it. But didn't seen concerned.

The breast nurse rang in the afternoon to see how I was getting on. I said that I was fine. I told her what the district nurse had said about the dressings, she asked if the district nurse had taken a swab. I said that she hadn't.

"We had better get you back in," She said. "Come into the clinic tomorrow at 2 o'clock and see the surgeon, the one who wears a bow-tie."

I thanked her and said that I would see her tomorrow.

I took Fred to the clinic to have his M.M.R. He was very brave. The nurse that did his injection was also one of the nurses that had looked after me in hospital. While we were there we saw the health visitor. She asked me why I had had my haircut. I told her the reason….She didn't take it very well.

October 28th

Felt exhausted today. Got up and had a bath. Went back to bed. Mum made me a lunch and then it was time to go to the hospital. I saw the surgeon and he waved at me. The breast nurse came in and we went into another room together. I took off my top and he examined me. He removed the dressings and said that they were healing well. He did notice that a lump had grown under my right arm. "If you go down to the breast clinic," he said "they will drain off some of the fluid which will make your arm easier to move." I thanked him and the nurse and I went downstairs. I was seen by a radiographer who used a scanning machine to pick up the lump. She sprayed on some of the pink spray and put in a needle, once that was in place she attached a syringe and drew out some of the fluid. She ended up collecting five 20ml syringes and one 10ml syringe full. "That should make it easier." she said. I thanked her and came home.

It feels much easier in my armpit now. My right arm is getting stiff and painful when I extend it. I must do some exercises. The top inside of my right arm is getting sorer.

Tonight it felt comfortable to lie on my side, so I snuggled up for a cuddle with Steve……nearly normal?………No.

October 29th

Helped with the boys this morning. Did my exercises, they hurt a little in the beginning but it got better. Did the ironing, had some lunch. Mum took the boys to the park. So I hoovered and polished. Feeling really fed up. I feel really frustrated because I can't do everything that I want to without something hurting. The trouble with me is that I am too impatient. I don't want to wait for nature to take it's course and make me better, I want to be better instantly.

October 30th

Exercises still hurts a lot. Given up, fed up. Went to see the healer. Feeling much better …calmer. I seem to be getting angry with everyone. The bolt things on the sides of me itch and catch whenever I lean over. It still hurts when I lift up Bill or Fred. Carried Fred upstairs for his afternoon nap today.

The children made their pumpkins tonight. We had a lovely, messy time, great fun.

At night my right hand, arm and leg twitch……it's a bit unnerving.

I spoke to my Mum and asked her if she had twitching in her arms and legs, she said that she did. That made me feel better. It's still weird though.

October 31st

Up early. F*** the exercises. I don't want to be around any one today.

Did the ironing. Helped with lunch. Bathed Bill and Fred. We put the pumpkins outside the front door. Someone stole Molly's one! Went to bed early at 9 o'clock and fell straight to sleep.

November

November 3rd

Had my post-operative two-week check today. I saw the surgeon with the bow tie. He said that the tumour had been 17mm in size and that they had taken out another one that had been behind it, that they did not see earlier. He said that they also removed eighteen lymph nodes and had found three of them had traces of the cancer in them..

The tears welled up again. He handed me some tissues. I had wanted to be told that the lymph nodes were clear. He reassured me that they had done their job by sieving out the cancer……I do hope that he is right.

I had an aggressive grade 3 negative breast cancer.

He took off the dressings. He said that they had healed well.

I looked down at them, they didn't look too bad. It was strange because all the time the dressings were on I thought that my boobs looked normal, just a bit covered up, but now they looked very flat with the nipples missing.

He told me that I could have stick on nipples. It made me smile, as I had a vision of Steve getting amorous and appearing with one stuck on his forehead.

As you can guess I declined the offer.

While I was there the surgeon put some saline into the right breast.

He got a large syringe full of saline and inserted the needle into the bolt under the right side. It felt cold as it went in, and slowly my boob began to grow.

When he had finished he told me that when they are filled to the brim they hold half a pint each.

He also told me that I would be getting an appointment with the oncologist in the next two weeks.

When I got home from hospital I started to get stabbing pains just above where they had put the saline in. I also had a throbbing headache. I took some paracetamol tablets and went upstairs to lie down. I felt really cold, so I decided to have a hot bath and then went to bed with a hot water bottle.

I couldn't sleep and it felt like I was waking up about every half hour.

November 4th

This morning Steve brought me up some breakfast, but the smell of it made me feel really bad. So bad in fact that I ended up being sick in the toilet. I got back into bed and felt freezing cold, but I was hot to the touch and sweating.

My index finger and thumb on both hands kept twitching and I couldn't stop shaking. I rang the hospital and spoke to one of the breast nurses. She said that it sounded like an infection and advised me to call the doctor. I did and arranged for the doctor to visit me at home.

Later in the morning the heath visitor came to see me, she said that there were organisations that would be able to help me with the children

33

when I was having treatments and didn't feel very well. She said that the one she would get in touch with for me was called 'Home Start'.

The doctor came round and took a look at me. She said that I had a chest infection and wrote out a prescription for some antibiotics, and some more iron tablets. She also talked to me about the chemotherapy and said that there were loads of different tablets for the sickness and if the ones that the hospital give me didn't work she would be able to offer alternatives.

My Mum had to get the coach home in the afternoon and Auntie Jill, our next-door neighbour came in to help until Steve came in from work. I got up to make tea for everyone and then I went back to bed. Slept loads and felt pretty rotten.

November 5th

Feeling much better. Going on holiday!!

When Steve came home from work we packed up all the children and went down to Hayling Island to Mill Rythe Holiday Park for a Fireworks Weekend. The children were so excited when we went through the gates, that it made it all worthwhile. It was half-board so that it wasn't long before we all sat down and had a nice meal with no washing-up! The children had loads of places to explore and different clubs to try out we didn't see very much of Jake and Molly.

November 6th

HAPPY BIRTHDAY ME!!!!

I opened my birthday presents and cards. I tried to be happy but all I felt was sadness. I cried while I was opening them, Molly asked if I was alright and I said that I was. It was that I was just so happy to be there with them all. I don't think that she believed me. She gave me a big cuddle.

I was crying because of the enormousy of my situation. As I sat there I found myself realizing that if I had not found the lump and they had not taken me seriously, (you hear lots of stories about women that keep going to the doctors with lumps and are sent away because they are told that it is nothing serious.) this could have been my last birthday.

Jake had a go at climbing a wall and made a new friend, so that was the last we saw of him. Molly went into the main hall and had a go at learning to samba! Bill and Fred went to play in a huge ball park. Steve and I? We just went with the flow. Tonight we have got a huge firework display and the entertainment is the 'Drifters' and a couple of comedians......just what the doctor ordered! They were all brilliant! The fireworks were fantastic!

November 7th
Came home.

November 8th
Got a letter from the hospital this morning; my appointment is on the 18th at 10:55am.

November 11th
Over done it today. I hurt all over. Taking painkillers.

November 12th
Under my arms is so sore. I've decided to do my Christmas shopping. I think that it will be a good idea because if the chemotherapy makes me feel yucky the last thing that I am going to want to do is fight the crowds at the shops.

November 13th
I can't pick up Fred today my sides are hurting, they feel as if they are bruised. It hurts across my left breast and under my right arm. Weight 8st 6lbs.

November 14th
I ache. All around my sides and across my chest. I know every one told me that I have been doing too much...... I have taken note.

November 18th
My first appointment with the oncologist. Dad came with me.
We sat in his office and he went through what was in the pathology report from my operation.
He told me that I would need chemotherapy because they cannot tell whether there is any cancer still inside me. He said that it is like

fighting an invisible army. You don't know whether they are there or not, but you cannot take that chance that they are not.

He said that the chemotherapy I would be having was called F.E.C. He wrote down the name of the drugs. He said that the one that begins with the letter E is the one that makes you lose your hair. He said that there are cold caps available and that they make the scalp cold which limits the amount of blood going to the hair follicles which in some cases stops the hair from falling out, so I could just have thinner hair. But, it may not work at all and I would end up bald. (I later found out that Swindon doesn't do cold caps.) The other thing it does is weaken the heart muscles, but he said my dosage was too small for it to have any affect!

The other two didn't have major side effects, but together they made you sick.

I could also end up with mouth ulcers, sore eyes, no periods (that one I can live with!), tiredness and I could start my menopause.

Fantastic I thought, not only will I become bald and throw-up but I will also be having hot flushes, mood swings and a sore mouth and all that over Christmas! What else could I ask for? He said that they would give me steroids and tablets to minimise the sickness and nausea. The chemotherapy ran on a twenty-one day cycle. For the first four days I would feel lousy, between seven and fourteen days my white blood cell level would be non-existent, they advised me that I didn't go in crowded places because of risk of infection, fourteen to twenty one days I will be normal. He said that if at any time I felt unwell I would have to get in touch with the hospital straight away, because I did not have the immune system to fight off infections without the help of antibiotics. He said that I had to be really careful.

I thought to myself that I should take Bill out of play-school because he was at the age when they pick -up all the bugs going round and then I was more than likely to get them as well. He also explained that how ever the chemotherapy affected me the first time is a good measure of how I would be all the way through. He explained that the cancer they had found was a junior version of the one in my Mum had. That sounded promising, as my Mum had beaten hers.

He said that mine was a negative one, but if I had been older, meaning menopausal age, that the cancer would have had a hormonal cell system, which would have reacted with tablets as well as chemotherapy.

He gave me the consent form to sign, which gave them permission to administer the drugs. He told us that the treatment would take an hour and a half. Two drugs would be put in with saline and the other one would be put in on it's own. He took us up to the ward where I would be having the treatment.

It was a strange, but all the people there looked as if they had cancer! They were all thin and most of them had no hair. They were hollow eyed and had black rings under there eyes. None of them smiled..... that would be me on Thursday, was all I was thinking........... How depressing.

The nurses seemed nice, one of them put her arm around me, I started to cry. They said that this was the hardest thing for anyone to cope with and they would be with me all the way. We went back to the oncologists office and confirmed the starting date. Thursday November 25th at 9 o'clock in the morning.

I was weighed, then they weighed Dad. They also measured me so that they could work out the amount of drugs needed. We said thank you and came home.

That afternoon I took Bill to see the doctor as he has developed a rash. The doctor says that he has got eczema and he gave me a prescription for some cream and some lotion to go in the bath with him..

While I was there I also booked myself in for a flu jab.

That night I sat down with Jake and Molly and read the leaflet that the oncologist had given me.

It had all the side effects and other bits and bobs that you needed to know about having the F.E.C. chemotherapy. They sat and listened to all the things that could happen, like me losing my hair and other things. "I suppose diarrhoea isn't too bad is it?" Jake said, after we had read it...... How simple life is to them!

November 19th

This morning I went to the doctors.(It seems like I am always either at the doctors or the hospital!)

The nurse that gave me a flu jab was the same one that gave Fred his M.M.R and looked after me in the hospital. I saw the doctor while I was there and told her that I was starting chemotherapy on Thursday. We had a nice chat and I also told her that I had thrush. She said that it was because of all the antibiotics that I have been given. She gave me a prescription to clear it up and an extra one just in case.

I have to remember to tell the nurse when they give me any injection or take blood from me that the can only use my left arm as the lymph nodes were removed from the right armpit.

November 21st

My cousin Darren and his wife Maeve came for lunch with their baby Jude today. We had a lovely time. We had partridge and pheasant that Jake got yesterday when he went beating. We had some bad news yesterday, our cousin Sharon, has passed away, at the age of 47. She had diabetes with complications.

November 22nd

Went shopping with Lucy for some head scarves in case my hair falls out.

November 23rd

HAPPY BIRTHDAY, MY DAD.

Took Steve to see "That'll be the day." at the theatre. It is a rock 'n' roll stage show with dancing, singing and comedy. It was absolutely fantastic! Just what we both needed . Weighed 8st 4lb.

November 24th

I had an appointment this morning with a woman at the advise centre as I had been told that I could be entitled to claim some benefits because of my illness. I was there for an hour and a half and she decided that the one we should try for was a disability allowance. We filled in all the forms and she sent them off.

In the afternoon I had an appointment with the surgeon who did my operation. He looked at the size of my boobs and decided that there was room in the right hand side for just a little bit more, he put in another 90ml. He said that they took 300ml in total (half a pint, just like the other surgeon said).

He said that the swelling under my left arm would go away in its own time. He also told me to feel underneath my left breast as there was a vein there that had protruded because of the swelling. It felt like a taut piece of string.

He didn't want me to be alarmed if I had felt it at any other time.

The breast nurse was also there and she said that she had a form for me that entitled me to have a wig made.

It had two addresses on; one was for a salon in town and the other one was for a lady who worked from home.

I decided that I would use the lady that worked from home at least I would have privacy and be able to take the children.

The surgeon said that he was very pleased with how I was doing and said he would see me again in six weeks.

As I was leaving he asked if I would take part in a project that they were doing in one of their departments in Southampton. It was interested in women who were forty and under with the same cancer as I had.

He said that they would use the data that had already been collected i.e. from the pathology report and other bits, but it would be helpful if I could fill in a questionnaire and let them take some blood from me.

On the way home I went into the chemist and picked up a form about pre-paying for prescriptions, as I would be paying for any medicines that I needed including my anti-sickness tablets. They gave me a phone number and I rang it when I got home.

I bought a certificate that lasted for four months and it cost of £33:41. I asked for it to start on the 25th.

Dad has brought me one of those knitted hats that have got pom-poms on and ear muffs with plaited wool straps that you can tie under your chin....He says that I can wear it when I have got no hair as it will keep my head warm. He thinks he is so funny!......I am never wearing it outside the front door........EVER!

Chapter 4

November 25th

D-DAY!!!

Chemotherapy session number 1. Mum and Dad came over early because I was going to have my chemotherapy at 9 o'clock. Dad and I went to the hospital. We were met by a lovely nurse.

There was also a woman from the W.V.R.S. who made Dad and I a cup of tea. They gave Dad a card to go in the window of the car because of the length of the treatment. It saves us putting more money in the machine.

The nurse sat down next to me and got a large pile of papers.

"Here we go!" she said. She went through what was going to happen, what drugs they were going to administer, why they were using those drugs in particular, the after-effects.......that was the thing that had been worrying me the most, mainly about being sick, and losing my hair.

I didn't realize that there were quite so many, lots more than we had been told previously.

The only one that seemed quite nice was that your skin can become darker, so maybe I will look like I have been on a very expensive winter holiday!

She then told me about the care I would need to give myself after having the treatments.

She gave me a thermometer and said that I would have to take my temperature every day. If it was 38' or over (it should be 37:4') I would have to be seen by doctor for antibiotics, if I wasn't taken seriously then I should come to the A & E department.

She gave me a card that I have to take everywhere with me. It says on it that I am having chemotherapy and what action was necessary if I was in need of medical attention. She also gave me a red book that had in it what drugs I was being given in my chemotherapy and all other prescription drugs that I was using in case anyone ever needed to know. Lastly she gave me a prescription for some anti-sickness tablets and some steroids to be picked up from the hospital pharmacy. (Good job I sent off for the pre-payment certificate.)

"Right." she said, "shall we start?" She went over to the desk and ordered the chemotherapy drugs, as they are made up individually.

She went to put a cannula in my left hand.

"We are nice to you and use children's ones, they are smaller."

The needle didn't sit in the vein properly. She had another go. And another go. And another go.

She then went and got some warm bags to put on my arm that should bring the veins up.

Another nurse then took over and put in the cannula. She hurt me.

She didn't have a back flow, which means the blood doesn't show when they pull back the syringe.

She had another go. BINGO! It worked! (I hate to think what mess they would of made of me if they hadn't used a child's size!) Poor dad, his hand had changed colour where I had been squeezing it.

Pain is all in the mind I could hear Steve saying to me. He always uses words like bananas or carrots if I was having something done that would hurt me, like having the drains taken out. At the moment they pulled, he would whisper in my ear. It made me smile thinking about it. But this time it was rubbish! This time it really hurt!

Maybe those words only work when Steve says it?

The nurse put on a pair of protective glasses as she administered the chemotherapy.

She had a drip running of sodium something to dilute the drug as it was going in. It went in through a junction coming off the line that was coming out of the cannula in my hand.

First she put in the contents of two syringes, one had steroids in and the other one had some anti-sickness in. She told me that they should work for the whole of the day and that I would not need to take any tablets when I got home.

"Ready?" She asked. "Yes, lets get it over and done with." I replied. Dad gave my hand a squeeze. I think he was more worried than me! First she put in two syringes of a red drug. They all had my name on and I had to say, yes, that was me. She told me it would make my wee pink for a while, I thanked her for this bit of information. She put the drug in ever so slowly and periodically she pulled the syringe back so that it filled with blood.

She did this so that it made sure that the drugs were going into my vein and not into any tissue as she said that it wouldn't be very nice.

She then put another syringe that held a clear drug. I also had to say that the name on it was me. Finally it was time for the last one that came in a bag that they hung up. It was covered in a silver bag, as the drug was light sensitive. It took about half an hour to go through. Once it had finished they put in a small bag of saline just to make sure that all the drugs had gone in and that there was none left in the line.

While the last one was going in my nose felt like it does if you have been swimming and you get some water up your nose. It feels like a sort of burning sensation, followed by a pain in your head. "That's normal." My nurse said. "Didn't I tell you that would happen?" "No." I replied. After it was all over we made an appointment for three weeks time. Dad went downstairs to the pharmacy and got the tablets that I needed to take home with me. They gave me a form so I could have a blood test done on the day before I was due my next treatment and we said good bye.

When we got home Mum suggested that she and Dad took Bill and Fred home with them so that I could see how I reacted to the drugs that I had been given.

So I packed a bag for them. After we had all had a cup of tea, I put the boys in the car. As I was putting the boys in those silly tears came back and I got myself in a right old state.

Dad gave me a huge cuddle and so did Mum. They got in the car and then they were gone.

Jake and Molly came home from school.

Molly and I went up to the vets to get the dog, Taz some worming tablets.

That night we had roast lamb for tea. I felt a bit dodgy but I thought that it was because I hadn't eaten very much in the day. After tea I still didn't feel any better. I was also very tired. When the children went to bed at 8 o'clock I went as well. I took two anti-sickness tablets, and a hot water bottle with me. I slept all night.

November 26th

Woke up starving! Had my breakfast and all the tablets that I needed to take, two steroids and two anti-sicknesses.

I felt all right, I felt normal.

Dad rang and asked how my night had been. I said o.k to both questions.

My Mum rang and asked the same thing.

I sent Jake and Molly off to school. I was alone in the house, it was a peculiar feeling. I hoovered, did the washing, cleaned the bathroom and then felt hungry, so I made myself an egg and bacon sandwich and took my next lot of tablets, two anti-sickness tablets.

I rang and arranged my blood test for the day before my next treatment, December 12th.

Had my tea, had some more tablets, two anti-sickness tablets.

As it was Friday night Steve went up the pub. I still felt fine so I walked up there with him, taking the dog. I came back home and did the ironing and had a banana, had the last tablets of the day, two steroids and two anti-sickness.

Went to bed .....exhausted. Weigh 8st 4lb.

BUT NOT FEELING SICK OR BEING SICK.

November 27th

Woke up and had my breakfast and my tablets. I feel all right but very drained, like I have no energy.

I read some of this diary it made me cry. I've been through so much but it just feels like a dream. It's like someone else is leading this life and I am only observing. It's only when I read it, does it become real. I still don't feel its me even though I can feel the physical pain. It is a very strange situation. These stupid tears won't go away, I'm so tired.

I decided that the only way to overcome this is to do something, so I changed the bed and put fresh linen on it. I had a bath. I then went back and laid on the bed. I felt better in the evening and made tea, then went to bed.

November 28th

Had breakfast and tablets. Feeling much better today. I went shopping with Steve for a suit as we have the funeral of his cousin tomorrow.

I have a bit of an upset stomach today. Had a lovely roast beef for lunch and after I went upstairs for a rest.

November 29th

God Rest Your Soul, Sharon.

Today was Sharon's funeral.

Funerals always make you feel very lucky to be alive, especially when it is the funeral of someone who wasn't very old.

Felt fine all day, took my tablets when I should.

November 30th

Very tired today. I pushed myself to get up and bathed. Went and got some frames to put the childrens school photos in. Came home and laid down. It took ages to put the shopping away. Noticed that I am so hungry today I can't stop eating.

Over did it, went shopping after tea to get some cold meat.

Steve had fallen asleep! He is no good to me. I had a cup of tea, it hurt my throat. Must keep an eye on that I thought!

December

December 1st

When I drank my tea this morning my throat was still sore. I checked my temperature it was normal.

The nurse had said that if you got a sore throat you should seek medical attention as you may have picked up a virus and your body is not as its best to fight it, so you may need antibiotics.

I had a bath. Got Jake and Molly up, scrapped the car, because it was covered with frost and we were at the A&E by 7:30am.

I gave them the little red book I had been given, the nurse then took my blood pressure, looked in my mouth and listened to my chest. They also took a gallon of blood.

The results? Blood count is fine. This is good, as I am starting my seven to fourteen day period.

They gave me some penicillin which I have to take for a week. The tablets have the most disgusting taste, they are absolutely gross. Steve said that it was good as it covers my dodgy week. Later I took Taz for a walk and posted some Christmas presents.

I may have acted irrationally by going up to the hospital, but the speech that they give you up at the hospital before you have your first chemotherapy treatment, does to an extent frighten you. They explain how poorly you will become if you do not pick up on any symptom or change and the fact that you may become hospitalised if they are ignored, so what are you to do? I have become a hypochondriac and monitor everything about myself, every day.

December 2nd

Bill and Fred are coming home!!

December 3rd

Back to normal, total chaos! We are finally ready to go and see the lady that would be fitting me with a wig.

I don't know what to expect. Is it made to measure? Is it off the peg? It's a thing that I don't really want to do. Old women wear wigs and they are so obvious that it is not worth having.

When we got to the ladies house she welcomed us in. She was ever so nice. She showed me some wigs, some have a micro-something bit on the top so you can see your skin through it. Others had a thick backing, they didn't look too bad.

We went through a book of styles to find one that looked like my hair now.

You choose three wigs that you like and they are ordered and then out of the three you choose the one that looks the best.

She also had lots of pieces of hair and we matched the best one with my hair colour. She said that they would be ready next week so we arranged a day and time and said goodbye. Bill and Fred were so good that I stopped at Burger King on the way home and bought them some chips as a treat. Came home and played trains. My period has started....lovely.

December 8th

The wig lady rang, the wigs haven't arrived. She will ring when they do.

December 9th

My head has become really itchy. When I scratch it bits of hair are coming out. I feel like a dog that is moulting, they leave hair everywhere.

December 10th

I can now pull clumps of hair out at a time. It makes you have a scary feeling inside. It's out of my control. But the strange thing is that I can't stop pulling it out. It makes it a reality that, yes, I am going bald and everyone is then going to know that I have got cancer.

People are going to look at me with pity in their eyes. Poor girl, she's got cancer. That is what they will be saying without words.....I hate pity.

Went to Mum and Dads for the first time since the operation. I had been looking forward to going it is something we did before cancer. It would make life feel back to normal or at least take my mind off going bald.

Steve shaved my head tonight. I look so ugly. A freak! I cried, I'd just got used to having no boobs and now I have no hair. Disgusting.

Fred woke up and I went in to settle him. He looked at my face and then my head. He had a confused look on his face and then he started to cry. I cried. Fred didn't recognize me.

I went to bed wanting to disappear and never be found.

December 11th

I wore a purple headscarf today.

47

I put it on before Jake and Molly saw me. I don't want them to see my head yet, not until I have got used to it.

We all went down to Hayling Island to visit Steve's Uncle and to give my Uncle his Christmas present. I also went to visit my Grandma's resting place and lay some flowers. I told her my news and fed the squirrels.

On the way home we stopped off at Dowies (Dowie or Dewie, as mum spells it, is Steves younger brother, he also has another brother, Andy, who is the youngest.) and got a Christmas tree.

It feels as if everyone is staring at me. I feel so different. It is so alien. I want this day to end. The first day out with something different about you is always the worst. Like when you went to school for the first time with your new Clarks shoes on and everyone used to point and snigger.

December 12th

Went to see the lady and have my wig fitted. My head is too small, she has got to send them back.

I feel really sick today.

Took some anti-sickness tablets...... Strange, why feeling sick today?

December 13th

Bill went back to play school today. They were really pleased to see him…and me. They said that I looked well, better than they thought.

Tonight we will put up the Christmas decorations. Twelve days till Christmas. I don't feel at all Christmassy.

December 14th

Tonight I flipped at Steve; there wasn't really a reason. I'm just fed up. I want to be how I was before I had cancer.. I don't want to have cancer any more. I want my breasts back with nipples and my hair back.

I weigh 8st 6lbs, which is my normal weight but I look absolutely awful with no clothes on. My ribs are sticking out. I've got those bolts things protruding out of my sides <u>AND</u> to top it all off, my pubic hair is coming out!

Everything is too much effort any more. I threw my dinner in the bin. Broke Jakes dinner plate.

Hit Steve, called him horrible names. Wanted him to go away. I wanted to shout and scream. I wanted to hurt someone. I wanted to cry, 'I hate being me.' I hate being restricted by this illness. I'm too tired to do much. But I'm not going to give up. It won't defeat me, it just makes me so sad. It's an ugly illness. It makes you feel and look ugly. I've got chemotherapy again on Thursday. More tablets. More restrictions on going out. More tiredness. Sickness. Illness. Sadness. Tears. Feeling ugly. Maybe tomorrow will be different....I doubt it. Nobody really understands.

December 15th

Went to the doctors early today to have my blood test for tomorrow.

I keep telling myself that the chemotherapy is good medicine and that it's making me better. It doesn't hurt or make you feel horrible. I think that it is working.

Positive thinking, that's what they call it, isn't it?

December 16th

HAPPY BIRTHDAY MY GRANDMA.

Chemotherapy session number 2.

The day started normally, but I was in a right fluster. I don't know why. I was telling myself that everything was all right that it was the last time, so there was no reason why this time should be any different.

But while I was busy getting the boys ready I was all fingers and thumbs. I was feeling all flustered and couldn't concentrate on anything. Mum and Dad came over and I got ready to go.

At the hospital we saw a different oncologist. He was very nice. He showed Dad and me my blood results on the computer screen. He said that there was a query to whether I could have the treatment as my platelets were only just over the basic.

(They were 1:54% and the minimum is 1:50%) But, after seeing me he said that he was happy for it to go ahead. He also wrote me out a prescription for enough anti-sickness, steroids and anti-sickness tablet, (different to the ones that I had last time as he said that these ones were more effective) to last until my treatments were finished. I ended up with a carrier bag full!

He also gave me a questionnaire to fill in which was a survey into younger women getting cancer. We said goodbye and Dad and I went along to the room for my chemotherapy.

We went into the room and this time we saw a different nurse. She was very nice and a better shot than the last one, as she only made one hole in me.

Everything was going fine until I suddenly felt extremely sick. Both the nurse and Dad must have seen the change in my face. The nurse shouted out "BUCKET!"

I felt awful..... I didn't want to be sick in front of all these people!

One of the nurses opened a window for me and I took some deep breaths.

Dad got me a glass of water. Thank goodness the feeling went away. They said that it had happened because the drugs had been put in faster this time and maybe with less saline.

The treatment didn't seem to last as long this time, or maybe concentrating on not being sick took my mind off it?

We made an appointment for the 6th January, and came home.

Mum and Dad took the boys home with them.

I cooked tea. I felt a bit sick but, no more than last time. I also really fancied a glass of coke so I did, it was delicious. I had my dinner and felt ever so tired so I curled up on the sofa.

I felt really small as if someone had shrunk me. I went to bed at 7 o'clock and felt very heavy. I couldn't even manage to put my pyjamas on. I started to cry, I felt so rotten. I took some more anti-sickness tablets because I started to feel sick again. I lay down, Steve came up and I didn't even have the strength to lift my head off the pillow. I fell asleep.

I woke at about 12 o'clock and had some more tablets, as I still felt sick. About half an hour later I was violently sick. It was horrible, but also frightening. Was it because they put the drugs in too quick or was it the coke?

December 17ᵗʰ

Went to the Co-op because I had a craving for a Pot Noodle. Spent most of the day resting on the bed. Felt sick, but more tired. I have got no interest in anything, no enthusiasm. I don't want to do anything.

December 18ᵗʰ

Woke up feeling a bit dodgy.

Spent the morning, washing and ironing. Jake went beating. The afternoon was spent upstairs on the bed. Still feeling sick but not as much as yesterday, just very tired.

December 19ᵗʰ

Feeling a bit better today, still feel sick. Maybe if I eat more?

Haven't been for a poo since Thursday, that's probably not helping. Went to the chemist and bought some suppositories. They worked o.k but not as good as they had in the hospital.

Steve cooked lunch it was delicious. Made some sandwiches for tea.

Felt very tired again, maybe tomorrow will be better.

I have noticed that my sense of smell has become more acute. On the kettle in the morning I can still smell Steve's deodorant and when Molly was in the back of the car I could smell the chocolate spread that she had spilt on her top. I can also smell the soap that people have wash with. It is a really strange thing to be able to do, it is almost like delving into their private lives.

December 20ᵗʰ

My stomach feels horrible, like there is a massive lump in there.

Used two suppositories, they worked a little bit more but still not enough. Ate some prunes, liquorice and oranges, something has got to get it going!

December 21ˢᵗ

Didn't work! Have rung the doctor. Got an appointment in the morning.

Had some Syrup of Figs.

Tania Bond

December 22ⁿᵈ

I went to see the doctor, she prescribed lactolose for my 'problem'. She also told me that all the things that I had taken would not have worked as they only aggravate the bowel, not stimulate it to work. I told her that I had got myself in a bit of a state when I went for my last treatment and I asked her if there was anything that I could take before I have the treatment to 'calm me down'. She said that she would write out a prescription for some Diazepam.

Went with Molly to see the lady about my wig.

She tried it on me but I didn't want to look in the mirror with anyone around. I wanted to see it on me, on my own without anyone there, just me, privately.

December 23ʳᵈ

Lactolose worked!!! I feel wonderful!!!

Bill and Fred came home.

Dad brought the turkey with him; it weighs 23lbs, the same as Fred!

Got a few mouth ulcers; keep catching them when I brush my teeth.

December 24ᵗʰ

I tried on my wig. Yuck! I looked weird with hair!

I don't think I will bother. Bill looks good in it. It looks like a Mullet on him. The wig lady came round and cut the children's hair and put some colours in Molly's. They all look fantastic.

December 25ᵗʰ

MERRY CHRISTMAS!

Didn't poo yesterday. Didn't this morning. My tummy is sore. Too much to do, not enough time to worry. Took lactolose.

The best bit of Christmas for me is to see the look on the children's faces when they come down in the morning and see all the presents under the Christmas tree. I love to hear the gasps and squeals that escape when they find their names on the presents under the tree.

Everyone was really pleased with their gifts, it makes it all worth while just to see the pleasure that they give.

Had a fantastic day, Mum and Dad came over. John and Lucy were also here. Everything was spot-on, food, presents, kids. Life was wonderful even without hair, boobs and being able to go to the toilet!

December 26th
Today I am very windy!

December 27th
Back to normal.
Today I showed Jake and Molly my head. I felt really sorry for them. Their faces showed a mixture of fear and revulsion all at the same time.
As soon as I had taken my scarf off I wished that I hadn't because as a mum you want to protect them from anything bad and this I had exposed them to myself. I asked them if they wanted to touch my head. The answer was.......no.

December 29th
Today we drove to Wales! We went to Caerphilly and didn't find a cheese shop!
Found some great puddles and rough roads to drive the Land Rover though.

December 30th
It feels wonderful to be doing normal things again. Today we went shopping. We spent ages looking round and then we lost Bill and ended up having all the staff and security people looking for him. We found him looking at all the pretty Christmas lights.
Johns friend Mark came down from Stoke for a couple of days.

December 31st
Lucy is going out to celebrate New Year tonight, she started getting ready at 3 o'clock!!!
Steve and I celebrated the other way...!
2005

January

January 1st
HAPPY NEW YEAR 2005!!

January 2nd
We all slept till 10 o'clock.

Dowie, Vicky, (Dowies daughter, our niece, she has a brother Vince.) John and Mark all joined us for lunch today.

I cooked a huge whole salmon, it was delicious. Watched Peter Kay video in the afternoon. Lucy and Mark went home today. Feeling fine but very tired.

January 3rd
Today we took all the Christmas decorations down. The house always looks so bare afterwards.

January 4th
Started my period. My eyes are all blurry.

I must start my arm exercises again as they are starting to get sore.

My breast nurse telephoned to see how I was getting on. I told her that I hadn't coped very well the last time I had chemotherapy, and that I had been to the doctors and she had prescribed some Diazepam.

The nurse listened and then suggested that instead of Diazepam I should have Loranzapam as it did the same, but it also had an anti-sickness effect as well. She told me to take one before I left for the hospital and then put another one under my tongue when they started to administer the drugs. She also gave me a list of mouthwashes and other bottles of stuff that would help me if I got mouth ulcers again.

Another piece of information she gave me was that when I was feeling sick to drink tonic water or ginger ale, as they both have quinine in, which is good for nausea.

Went to the doctors to have my blood test. I asked if there was a doctor available to see as I had some things that I would like on prescription that the breast nurse had advised me to have.

I waited a while and one of the other doctors saw me and said that it wouldn't be a problem for me to have any of the items; he also, complimented me on my headscarf.

January 5th

Jake, Molly and Bill start back to school.

I don't wear my head scarf when I am indoors, I go 'alfresco!'

I think that one of the worst parts of this illness, or the treatment is losing your hair. It is not a vanity thing, it is a confidence matter.

If you are going out and your hair doesn't go right, your day is ruined.

If you go out and you have no hair to 'go right', you day is always ruined. Even if you do wear a colour co-ordinated hat or scarf!

I also have another, I don't know how to describe it, it is like a physical taste. It is like the sensation that you have when you eat peanut butter, your mouth becomes almost dry and your tongue gets stuck on the roof of your mouth when you try and clear it, but you also have a taste similar to peanut butter. It is very strange as I haven't had peanut butter for years.

January 6th

Chemotherapy session number 3.

I wasn't as nervous today as last time; I kept thinking to myself that my blood count would be too low and that they would send me home early.

I had also taken one of the tablets that the nurse had suggested.

This time was saw another oncologist, (the top bloke!) my blood count was 1:76 which was much better than last time.

As I sat down to have my chemotherapy I put one of tablets under my tongue. They gave me my anti-sickness in tablet form this time rather than intravenously. The nurse also made sure that there was more saline going in the same time as the drugs. This time the whole thing was much better. We arranged the next treatment for the 27th. When we got home I felt fine.

The boys went home with Mum and Dad. I had something to eat, had my tablets and went to bed.

Steve came up at 10:30pm, I had some more tablets and I slept through until the morning.

January 7th

Woke up feeling fine. Took all my tablets.

Steve had the day off and I spent most of the day on the sofa watching television. I felt a bit sick, but mainly I felt really flat.

January 8th

No good to anyone. Spent the day in bed feeling rubbish. I felt sick and so tired, exhausted from the inside out.

Steve cooked tea, fish fingers and chips. Got up at 8 o'clock in the evening and had a bath. Changed my pyjamas and got back into bed......But I think my hair is starting to grow. Fantastic!

January 9th

Got up early, and put the meat in for lunch. Did the ironing, rang Mum and Dad to see how Bill and Fred were. They were still asleep.

Did the vegetables and then had an energy spurt. Bacon sandwiches, tablets and then I cleaned the kitchen from top to bottom. John came for lunch.

Feeling nearly normal.

Started using a mouthwash as my mouth is beginning to fall apart. It tastes disgusting!

My boobs are starting to look quite nice.

Especially the right one. All the bruising and swelling has gone. The left one is still a bit bigger underneath.

After lovings I noticed bruises on the inside at the top of my thighs. I wouldn't mind but it looks like someone has been nasty to me.

My exercises have helped my arms a lot.

Half way through the treatment, maybe there is a light at the end of the tunnel?

January 10th

Cried today. It seems like I haven't cried for ages, I don't know why. It happens when Steve leaves for work and I am on my own and the little'uns are still asleep.... thinking time, not good.

Finished another lot of tablets today. Tomorrow I am off them completely....No not really, only till the next chemotherapy session.

Nearly normal, I'm always saying that, soon it will be true. I feel fine, just not me. After this I will properly have to 'find' myself. Maybe the new me will be different. Not too different, maybe kinder, more patient, loving? We will have to wait and see.

Did the garden today. Re-potted everything in the greenhouse. Tidied up the front. How wonderful, I totally lost myself.

I haven't had trouble going to the toilet this time as every night I have taken some senakot. I didn't want the same problem as I had the last time that was horrible. Finished the anti-sickness tablets that 'bung' you up today. Will take one senacot tonight and that should do it. I weighed 8st.10lbs.

I have noticed that I look bigger across my shoulders and neck and that my clothes seem tight across my bust. Maybe it's the steroids? I hope I don't end up looking like a body builder?

I brought myself a new long sleeved tee shirt.

It's strange because I am not that big, only 5ft 3ins but had to buy a top sized 16! Vince passed his driving test today at 3:30pm, who's a clever boy then!

January 11th

Feel shit.

January 12th

Brought some Bio-Oil today; it's supposed to reduce scars. Lets see.

After my bath I noticed my eyes start to do funny things. It looked like a large question mark made out of a kaleidoscope. I haven't had one of these for ages. The doctor told me that they were 'visual migraines'. It lasted for half an hour and then I had a thumping headache. That made me feel brilliant as I was still feeling sick anyway. My legs felt as if they are full of jelly and my head feels like it is a washing machine. Ho-hum. Never mind, eh?

January 13th

My head is still throbbing and I feel rubbish. I didn't get up when I should this morning.

We all went to the dentist. She felt around my jaw, face and throat, don't know why, she must do though.

Spent the afternoon with Jake and Molly; feeling so much better. Sickness has gone…..for the moment.

Mum and Dad brought Bill and Fred home this afternoon.

January 14th

Feeling normal! Busy day. Felt slightly dizzy a couple of times, life is better.

Brought a new washing machine today, got ten pounds for the old one. It was only good for spare parts! Went out walking with Bill, Taz and Fred.

Bill said that the trees haven't got any leaves.

It made me think about my head, bare like the branches on the trees.

I thought that when the trees get their leaves in the spring, it should be about the same time as I get my hair back. How philosophical!

Had a long chat with the Health Visitor this afternoon, she came round to check up on us. She is straight talking and down to earth. We put the world to rights, well for the afternoon at least.

January 16th

I'm feeling really down today; I don't trust Steve. I think he has or will find someone else.

I don't blame him. I've got no hair. I've put on weight, 8st 11lbs.

I'm moody, I shout at the kids, I feel so ugly.

I'm not at all attractive to look at or know.

Maybe I should go. Fat ugly bitch!

January 18th

Steve asked me this morning if I wanted him to come home tonight. I told him it was his home.

How can someone love you when you don't love yourself? If he didn't love me it wouldn't matter.

I think it would make me feel better if he thought that I was fat and ugly too. My clothes don't fit and my neck and shoulders look like they belong to a weight lifter. How can he love me when I look like this?

When he met and fell in love with me, I was healthy, thin, had long blonde hair and I felt beautiful, sexy and so wonderful.

Now because I have no nipples or breasts loving is just not the same. So, I'm not going to bother. There in no point. If it doesn't make you feel WOW, have it as a fantastic memory of the old life before cancer destroyed everything that made my life mine.

Steve kept on to me tonight asking what was wrong. We had a long chat. He made me cry. I needed to cry. It's a pain deep down inside, it's a grief for my old life.

My simple life. My old life. I was a mum, a wife, and a daughter.

I got up in the mornings and did what I had to do and then went to bed in the evening. Simple.

Then that life was taken away. It's no longer my life. Cancer rules this life. Treatments and side effects live my days. I look in the mirror and the person looking back isn't me. I've gone away. I hope I can come back soon. Maybe it's a way of coping. Some people would call it denial.

I call it survival. I will survive and come out the other side, I just need some help and without Steve I don't think that I would be able to do it.

Lucy has come down for the weekend.

January 15ᵗʰ

Man has come to mend the tumble dryer, he is sending some new bits in the post.

January 17ᵗʰ

We have a pair of Blue Tits in the garden, they are checking out the nesting boxes in the Cherry tree.

January 19ᵗʰ

Went to Coate Water with Bill and Fred. We walked around the lakes. It's the first time since my operation. That's got to be a good sign, hasn't it?

Molly has had all her beautiful hair cut off. There are loads of cases of nits going around the school and it will be easier for her to look after.

January 20th

Today I had an urge to do loads of baking; pastry, steak and kidney pie, bread pudding and custard. Went to bed very tired.

January 21st

Went with Bill and Fred to Mum and Dads.

Lucy came down for the weekend.

Noticed a red rash around where my nipple would have been on the left breast at bedtime.

January 22nd

The red rash is still there but not so prominent. Feeling better about myself. Weighed myself 8st 9lbs.

Molly was sick in the night. Fred was sick after tea. Hope it's just them or I expect they will postpone my chemotherapy on Thursday because I won't be well enough. It's snowing!

January 23rd

Bill wore 'big boy' pants all day, no accidents! Lazy day, big roast beef lunch.

Terry came round in the afternoon with a brace of pheasant. He also said that he would be taking Jake again with him the next time he went.

January 24th

Bill's at play school today, took Fred to the 'foot clinic', he is being referred.

Auntie Jill, came in for a cup of tea. I gave her a hyacinth.

Today was a good day.

January 25th

Steve isn't very well today, he spent the day in bed. Fred has got a nasty cold, I'm glad that I had a flu jab.

January 26th

Had my blood taken. Everyone at the doctors said how well I looked. They asked how I was getting on.

It took the nurse a long time to find a good enough vein.

They said that coughs and colds don't affect your blood count, so maybe tomorrow will go ahead as planned.

Steve is still poorly in bed. Bill has now got a cold.

Good job I haven't got a serious illness, isn't it!

I keep shouting at Jake and Molly, I know it's not their fault, well it is really, they don't listen. Everyday I say the same things and they just don't take any notice. Maybe I haven't got as much patience as I usually have or as much energy. Maybe I usually follow behind, picking up, tiding up, putting away robotically without thinking and maybe because I'm ill and don't have as much energy and patience, things are more obvious. Maybe I am losing my mum skills?

I have such low self-esteem. I feel that I am at the bottom of the pecking order, the lowest of the low. If I was living in Medieval times even the lepers would be royalty compared to how I feel.

January 27th

Chemotherapy session number 4.

Weight now 8st 11lbs. Disgusting but can't shift it.

Steve is still in bed, not well.

Dad and I arrived at the hospital and were called in straight in. My blood was better this time, it can go ahead. I told the doctor that I was taking an extra anti-sickness tablet on the night of the chemotherapy and now I wouldn't have enough to last till the last treatment. He wrote out a new prescription. I also told him that I had been getting nasty stomach aches. He asked me to lie on the couch and he felt and listened to my abdomen.

He said that everything seemed fine down there. While he was there I showed him the bruises on my thighs. I think that I shocked him; he wasn't expecting to see that part of me.

He said that it was unusual to have bruising there but it was caused by the change in blood cells.

Nothing to worry about. I asked him about the radiotherapy. I didn't know if it was dangerous to Fred, like the bone scan I had earlier.

He was surprised that we didn't know all about it. "Weren't you told this when you signed the consent form?" He asked. "No." I replied. "We only signed for chemotherapy not the radiotherapy.""Oh." He said. He looked at my records. I hadn't been booked in. "We had better get this organised." He suggested. He told us that because I needed more surgery on my breasts it was not possible to have the treatment every other day. It would be daily for five weeks. The first time I go there they will measure me and put two tattoo marks on my breasts so the machine knows where to work.

He said that there were some side–effects; tiredness, sunburn and a rash that could blister and weep…nice!

He suggested that I started rubbing cream like E45 onto the area which would soften the skin and so reduce any reaction. He also said that because the radiotherapy touches the chest wall there is a chance that if it touches my lungs I could develop lung cancer, but he said that they were talking in terms of decades, not any time soon.

I'm not too concerned because I need the radiotherapy to finish off my treatment for this cancer. Also I will be going for so many check-ups that if I were to develop something I shouldn't they would be able to pick it up straight away.

The doctor filled in the consent form. I signed it. He said the treatment should start in about four weeks after the chemotherapy had finished. We went down to have my chemotherapy. We saw another new nurse and we were in a side room. She made Dad sit apart from us. She didn't ask me to check the labels and she didn't wear the special glasses. We had a nice chat and I told her that my hair was growing. She suggested that I shaved my head again and cream it every day.

Creaming would bring my hair through thicker. She said that the hair that I had at the moment was thin and patchy, as pure blonde hair doesn't fall out. So that is why my new hair looked wispy and fine!

The chemotherapy went smoothly, actually I fell asleep. I think that Dad got a bit bored. When we got back, mum and dad took the boys home with them.

We had poached cod, vegetables and new potatoes for tea . I felt very sleepy while I was eating and after I went straight to bed. I took an anti-sickness tablet and went to sleep at 6 o' clock.

Granddad Bond has been taken into hospital.

January 28th

Steve is better today, he has gone to work.

Felt fine this morning. Had a bath and shaved my head. It feels really shiny and smooth.

Went to the chemist and brought some E45 to put on my head and my breasts. Sitting on the sofa my head kept on sticking to the back of it. Instead of gliding across the leather it judders.

I took two senakot tablets at bedtime.

Granddad Bond is still in hospital.

January 29th

HAPPY BIRTHDAY IAN.

Feeling fine. Normally Saturday is the worse day for being tired, but not this time. Took all the tablets.

They are saying that Granddad Bond has got Parkinson Disease and Pneumonia?

January 30th

Woke up feeling fine.

Started to get nasty stomach acid. It happens every time. I have also worked out what the funny taste is in my mouth.

It reminds me of seawater when you have been in the sea swimming and later you taste it on your fingers.

That is the taste this medication gives me.

January 31st

Feeling really sick today. I know deep down I won't be, so I go into town. I always carry a plastic bag with me, just in case. But if I was ever sick out I would die with embarrassment. Feeling better now, going out takes your mind of it as you are busy thinking of other things.

Got nasty stomach cramps as well. Never mind it doesn't last forever.

Had some tonic water with a twist of lemon. It really works, feeling much better.

Steve has hurt his back at work today.

February

February 2ⁿᵈ

My period has started. It's really heavy this month.

No wonder I've been such a grouchy cow.

Poor family. I would hate to live with me.

My mood swings are getting worse. I seem to feel really angry and can't stop being rude to people no matter who they are, even Fred is getting the same treatment. I know while I am saying nasty things that there is no reason for it, but I can't seem to be able to stop saying them.

My hair is growing nicely, but very see-through.

Steve reckons that it is about 2mm long. Not bad for four days growth.

I've had headaches for the last three days and my throat is starting to get sore when I drink hot drinks. It's quite comforting to have the same symptoms each time because you can judge roughly when you will feel better.

This time after the chemotherapy I fancy chocolate ovaltine. After the last treatment it was hot water and lemon in it, the treatment before it was grapefruit juice! It's like being pregnant and having cravings.

My arm is still sore from Thursday. It feels really stiff inside like there is a metal pole in there stopping it moving. When I went shopping on Sunday I couldn't stretch to reach the top shelf and had to ask for some help. My left palm has also become very itchy, which is no good seeing as the saying goes, left leaving, right receiving.

What am I going to lose now?....

MY PUBIC HAIR!!

Shaved off the rest of it as there were only twelve left and they looked very sad.

It is much tidier now.

John is not very well now, even more pleased that I had that jab!

February 3ʳᵈ

Molly had the orthodontist today, they want to see her again in a years time.

Period is even heavier today. I had an accident and had to change my clothes. I haven't done that since I was a teenager.

Had to shave under my arms. I had so much hair! I am so happy and excited, rang Mum to tell her. Steve just gave me the 'look' when I told him. He never gets excited about anything!

The boiler broke down today. No water or heat.

No change with Granddad Bond.

February 4ᵗʰ

Boiler is fixed!

It is amazing how reliant you become on certain things, like running hot water.

February 5ᵗʰ

Throat is really sore today.

Having trouble going to the toilet again, took two senakot.

This morning all around my hair line it felt like I was sweaty, but I touched it and it felt fine. My legs also feel wobbly and my hands have been shaking.

I think that I need something to eat so I made some lunch.

I took my temperature, 37:7'. I rang the breast clinic and explained how I felt; she said that it sounded like low blood sugar. I told her that I had felt better after eating and that my period was heavier than normal. She said that all that plus being in my middle week would cause these symptoms. She said to keep an eye on my temperature and that if it went down to ring the hospital and ask for a blood test as I might have a viral infection.

My scars seem to be getting fainter since I have been using the Bio-Oil. Not all of the scar though, at the outside edges it is quite thick and purple, the Bio-Oil has made no difference at all to that bit.

I also have no feeling on the skin that is over the implants. If I run my finger over my my stomach and up to my neck I can feel it all the way but the implant bits I can feel the pressure of my finger but not the sensation. Does that make sense?

It is hard to describe and put into written words, sorry.

February 6ᵗʰ

Temperature has gone up and I feel better today. Also going to the toilet better.

My left arm has a bruise that has bumped; it is still very sore….Me? I feel fantastic and have got loads of energy.

Changed all the beds and did the washing. Made roast chicken for dinner.

Sorted out the garden and washed the windows.

Made a cake and had a lovely tea.

Bathed all the children and now writing this.

My hair is still making me feel really happy inside. Growing beautifully. Normality is returning.

I'm still finding loving difficult. My breasts and nipples were so sensitive and always played a big part. When Steve kisses or holds me the shivers and tingles are still there just the same as they always were, but, they only travel so far and then stop. It makes me sad. When something works that well you never try it any other way and now that way is gone.

I just don't know where to start and find a new way to make the magic……. spark?

Granddad Bond is getting better, he is eating and is awake more. Good news!

February 7th

Somehow last night the spark returned as a huge firework! Maybe writing things down really does help.

February 9th

My Mum has come down to stay for a couple of days.

Feeling lost and a bit down. Doing lots of daydreaming and sighing. I think that because Mum is here it takes the pressure off me because it changes the role I play. I have been demoted. I should be glad that someone else is 'being mum', but all it does is give me time to dwell and that is not healthy. Took Fred to the Bio-mecanics Clinic. They say that his feet are fine, but will see him again in six months time.

February 10th

Jake, Molly and Bill have broken up from school.

Did you know that you can lose all your body hair except the hair on your legs? I brought an eyebrow pencil and some false eye lashes in case I lost them, but I was very lucky, I didn't.

All I lost is the hair on my head, armpits and pubic area. All! It makes it sound so matter of fact written down. When it happens it is terrible, but it is amazing how you adapt to different things in your life. I don't give it a second thought putting my scarf on before I go out the door.

Auntie Dor has been taken into hospital, so has Uncle Johnny.(mums sister and her husband.)

So many people are unwell.

February 11th

Health Visitor came today, just to check up on me. She doesn't come in her professional capacity, she comes as a friend.

Uncle Johnny has come home from hospital.

February 12th

Fred took 2 steps today!

I find myself looking at people's hair. I am amazed that they go out with greasy hair, sometimes it's not even brushed.

I think it is because I haven't got any of my own, but I keep thinking to myself. 'If I had hair that long I would wear it up rather than leaving it all scraggy, or, I would never go out with roots that colour!' It is true what they say, you don't miss it until it's gone.

Auntie Sylvia came down to spend the day with us. She said that she was surprised how well I looked. I think that people have an image of how you should look when you have cancer and when you don't resemble that image they are always surprised, pleasantly, I hope.

February 13th

My Mum went home today.

February 14th

Valentine Day. Present? Card? Flowers?.............

Behave. Normal day, he says. He says he tells me that he loves me every day so why line the pockets of commercial money makers!

Tania Bond

February 15th

I am so tired. It seems that I get up, wash, get the little'uns ready, give them their breakfast and then all I want to do is go back to bed. This feeling lasts all day and gets worse in the afternoon. Poor me. If only I could sleep in a soft bed for a couple of hours, trouble is the little'uns would find me and want to play.

Fred can roar like a lion!

February 16th

Tiredness is getting worse.

The nurse couldn't find a vein today when I went for a blood test. She made me cry. I think that I have just had enough. She gave me a cuddle and told me that I was doing brilliantly.

Getting ratty with the children.

Being tired makes me less patient than I normally am, it also makes me feel a bit sick. Tiredness makes me feel sick. I wouldn't be tired if I wasn't having chemotherapy, chemotherapy makes me feel sick. Everything makes me feel sick. I can't even drink coffee any more, that makes me feel sick, too much tea makes me feel sick. I only have one cup in the morning 'cause it makes me feel sick. I now drink them herbal teas, especially ones with ginger......to help with feeling SICK!

Took Bill and Fred for a walk in the country, went with Auntie Jill and her dog Trudy. Found loads of flowers that are out early;

cowslip, daffodils, snowdrops and loads of tree blossom. Fed the ducks. It helped a bit. Nature does cheer you up.

Fred head-butted me tonight when I was getting him ready for bed, he didn't mean to. It made me cry and topped off the day.

February 17th

Chemotherapy session number 5.

'One more to go!'

Went to see the oncologist. My blood count is low, 1:01. It should be 1: 5 or over. He suggested coming back on Monday. I asked if it was worth having another blood test today. He said that it could but he would be very surprised if it made any difference. Dad and I went down to the department and had another test done. There was a huge waiting room full of people. It took forty-five minutes for us to be seen.

Result! My new blood count was 1:94, I could have my chemotherapy. We had to wait to be seen and eventually we went in.

Dad and I sat next to a lady that we usually just say 'Hello' to. She is lovely. She made us laugh.

She was with her son who plays rugby for Swindon.

The chemotherapy went well, although I did feel rather sick, but, because we were talking the whole time it didn't make it as noticeable.

We got home at 5 o'clock; we had been at the hospital since 10:45am.

Steve was home from work and had already given the children their tea.

Mum and Dad took the boys home with them. We had our tea, and I went to bed at 6:30pm. Woke up when Steve came to bed and had an anti- sickness tablet. Slept through.

Weighed …..8st 13lbs.

Fred is walking beautifully.

John brought me a pink breast cancer bracelet.

Auntie Dor is home from hospital.

February 18th

Feeling better. Had breakfast and all my tablets.

Exhaustion hit me. I lay on the bed and couldn't even lift my head. I just looked at the ceiling. It is such a weird sensation having no energy.

It has started snowing.

February 19th

HAPPY BIRTHDAY JAKE!

He is at his Grandmas. Good job that he is away as I feel the same as yesterday.

They said that I would feel tired but this is awful, even going downstairs makes my legs feel like jelly and my head all spinney. Went back to bed.

It is not a true tiredness; you lay with your eyes shut, but you just lay, you don't sleep. It is snowing.

February 20th

Feeling much better. Sunday lunch as normal. Jake and Molly came home. Made Jake a trifle with candles on. Went to bed at 8 o'clock, at least I stayed up all day.

It is still snowing.

February 21st

Jake and Molly are back at school. Got up and went to town. Snowing again.

February 22nd

Feeling like I did at the weekend. Steve had an appointment at the hospital for his leg. Molly had Brownies. Steve had an appointment at the chiropractor. Jake is being really nice?

February 23rd

Molly had a football match...they lost 3-0.

Vince has gone to Barcelona to watch Chelsea play. They went over there with no tickets and couldn't get any so they watched on a television.

February 24th

My boys are home. Chaos.

More snow.

February 25th

Normal, no tablets. No feeling sick.

Snowing again. Went for a walk with Bill, Fred and Taz. Came home and did painting, gluing and cutting up, made a lovely mess.

Felt a bit tired in the afternoon but doing fine. Hair is still fantastic, looks a bit grey in colour maybe I should change my name to 'The Silver Fox?' Lucy is down for the weekend.

Found loads of ants in the kitchen! It's February!! Going to see Granddad Bond tomorrow, it's not looking too good again.

February 26th

Went to the hospital to say 'Goodbye' to Granddad Bond, he isn't awake. He looks so tiny, you want to put him in your pocket and take him home. It reminds me of visiting my dad.

God Bless.

Snowing again, still settling.

March

March 1st

Hurt my back yesterday, visited the chiropractor this morning. She said that she could not treat me the same as she normally did because I was having chemotherapy. She had a good go anyway and made my back feel a lot better.

My period had also decided to arrive today, no wonder I feel so yucky. It seems like I am always having periods. My cycle has changed from being once a month to having one ever three weeks. They said that it would change my cycle, but they led me to believe that it would decrease and maybe stop, not increase so I was having more and that they would become heavier and the P.M.T would become worse!

My wisdom teeth have also decided to play up and are throbbing, beautifully.

I'm not coping very well today. Bill and Fred are driving me nuts. I'm so tired and all they want to do is play with me. They won't leave my side. Fred is using me as a climbing frame!

Bill decided to climb onto the windowsill when I was making their lunch and he knocked over the huge pot which smashed and split dirt all over the carpet. It made a huge mess everywhere. I just want to be left alone. It was the longest day ever.

Bedtime took so long to arrive.

Dowie rang this evening. Granddad Bond died this afternoon.

March 2nd

Every night I have been covering my hands in great dollops of E45 because they are so dry.

I told the nurse on the telephone. She told me that the chemotherapy was causing the dryness.

She said that the dryness was coming from the inside out and putting cream on wasn't really helping. She said that I needed some tablets. She said to get some called Pyridoxine and to take three, three times a day. She told me that the proper name for the dryness was Planter Palmer Erythema; she also added that alcoholics suffer from the same condition.

I went to the doctors this morning to arrange a time for my blood test, I asked for a prescription for some of these tablets.

March 3rd

Picked up the tablets, let's hope that they work.

Molly is spending the day up at New College.

March 4th

Awful rain today, Steve was home from work early.

March 5th

Today when we woke up there was thick snow everywhere. Jake, Molly and Bill went out into the garden and were playing snowballs and skidding on the ice. I took some video of them.

The snow doesn't seem as good as it was when I was little. I remember it laying so thick that you had to dig yourselves out of the house. It used to be so thick we couldn't get to school. Now you are lucky if it's an inch thick.

March 6th

Steve came home from the pub last night and decided to run a bath, but, went to bed before it had finished!!! When I got up the bath was overflowing hot water, the floor in the bathroom was soaked and downstairs my kitchen resembled a swimming pool! There was water running down the walls and over the counters, just like waterfalls. It had even reached the carpet in the front room.

Happy Mothers Day to me.

Guess what I spent the day doing?

I did get some nice slippers though.

March 9th

Bill came home from nursery and announced that it was very, very nice there.

March 10th

Chemotherapy session number 6.

Dad rang this morning and asked if Auntie Jill could look after the boys as Mums sister, Auntie Dor was ever so poorly and she needed to go and be with her..

I rang the hospital and asked if it was possible to postpone my treatment to next Thursday rather than today. I explained that we had the funeral of our Granddad on Tuesday and that our auntie was also very poorly.

The nurse that I spoke to said she would have a word with the oncologist and ring me back with an answer.

As it turned out my blood count was much too low for me to have my treatment today anyway, it was 0:88. They said that the oncologist would have preferred me to have my treatment on Monday, but because of the circumstances he would allow me to wait a week as long as I went on some antibiotics.

They told me the name of the tablets and I rang the doctors. They made it up in a prescription for me to go and collect. In the afternoon I felt really down. This would of been my last chemotherapy.

I had been excited in an odd way.

It was going to be the end of the nastiest chapter in my life. I kept crying and not being able to concentrate. Everything seemed to be happening in slow motion. I want to be on my own.

Everyone is telling me not to worry, that it's only a week and that it would go really quickly.

I knew that it was true, but that wasn't the point.

It should have been over today. The side–effects should have been over by next week, not just starting. Nobody understands what it is like and now the end has been postponed.

March 11th

Dowie rang this morning, Auntie Dor died at 12:30am.

God bless her and keep her safe.

March 13th

My hair now looks and feels like Action Man's!

I am nearly brave enough to go out without my scarf. I know that the first time you do something it is the worst, but I don't think that I can do it just yet.

March 15th

Granddad funeral, God bless your soul.

It was a sad, but lovely day.

March 16th

Had my bloods done. Hopefully for the last time. She said that all my veins had gone very deep and she had trouble finding one.

She hurt me but I didn't cry this time.

When I went to go she gave me a big hug.

"See you soon." she said…..I hope not!

March 17th

HAPPY BIRTHDAY JOHN!

My last chemotherapy!

Dad and I went to the hospital; the weather was ever so windy. I was quite glad that I didn't have any hair for it to mess up, Dad looked a right state! We got there just in time. The oncologist said that my bloods were fine and the last treatment could go ahead. I told him that I had been getting a pain on the left side of my pelvis.

He asked if my bowels were all right. He asked about my periods and I told him that they had become heavier and more frequent. He asked me to lie down so that he could feel where the pain was. He said that he couldn't feel anything wrong but he would send me for a scan to check that there was nothing there that shouldn't be, for instance fibroids. While we were there he rang up to find out about the radiotherapy, they could not give an exact date but it would be in about five or six weeks.

He asked for a urine specimen to rule out an infection and said that if there was a problem that I would be informed by my G.P.

He then stood up and shook dad and my hands.

"How do I know if this has worked?" I asked. "We don't." He replied. "But we will keep an eye on you and every three months you will be seen either by us or the surgeon"

We said our goodbyes and left.

Outside his office one of the nurses gave me a bottle to 'do the honours'.

When I came out Dad was trying to sell one of the nurses a car! We went into the room for the chemotherapy and the nurse who first gave me my treatment called us over and was already and waiting.

It made me feel that Dad and I were really liked.

I sat down and she began. She put the needle in and tried to get the back flow to check that it was sitting in the vein properly, there was no blood so she gave it a wiggle, it did an 'alf hurt!

I squeezed Dads hand, the blood showed.

I took an anti-sickness tablet and the treatment began. The lady who's son played for Swindon sat next to me and soon we were all having a right old natter. The chemotherapy was over ever so quickly. We said goodbye and thank you.

We came home. Mum and Dad took the boys home.

I was alone. I felt strange. It's over but I didn't feel any different. No different to last week or last month, before the operation or last year before we knew anything. I should feel happy that it is over, but I don't. I don't feel sad either. I'm indifferent.

It should be a significant moment, the end of chemotherapy, but in reality it is just another day.

Just another Thursday.

John came round for his tea. He had his presents and his cake. We sang him Happy Birthday. I took my tablets and went to bed.

Chapter 5

March 18th

Woke up feeling fine. The sun is shinning. Cut the grass and put the washing out on the line to dry first time this year. Felt 'normal' all day.

March 20th

Still feeling fine. Don't understand.

I don't feel sick or tired. Maybe it is because I had an extra weeks gap between treatments, or maybe it is because I haven't got to have anymore chemotherapy?

March 21st

Today Auntie Dors funeral. God bless her soul. The service was beautiful. Everybody was there.

She was buried in a plot near to Sharon so that they would always have company and never be alone.

Felt fine but after the service I got an awful pain in my pelvis, this time it was on the right hand side. It made me cry. It only lasted a short while, then went away.

March 22nd

Having awful trouble going to the toilet. Have taken some senakot and lactolose but they don't seem to be helping.

Rang and organised my pelvis and abdomen scan, booked for April 11th at 12:15pm.

March 23rd

After going to the toilet this morning I noticed a small amount of blood at the end.

Got a letter from the hospital asking me to telephone and arrange my scan?

March 24th

Still fine. Not feeling sick or tired.

Everyones last day, Steve from work and the children from school. Easter Holiday has begun.

Now going to the toilet as normal. Maybe I had over strained and caused myself to bleed?

Got a letter from Oxford with a huge list of dates for my radiotherapy sessions.

My first meeting is on the 6th April. I start my treatment on April 27th.

March 26th

Steve and I went to Oxford and timed it. It took fifty minutes, door to door.

Took the children to Coate Water, found loads of frogs. Jake had taken his wellies off because they had filled up with water and when he went to put them on again a frog was hiding in the toe and he nearly squashed it, yuck!Got absolutely filthy, we all had a bath when we got home. Brilliant fun.

March 27th

Started my period.

March 28th

My period is very painful this time. It is not like this normally.

March 30th

HAPPY BIRTHDAY VICKY.

Raining.

I have no patience with Bill and Fred today.

Everything that they do is annoying me. It feels like there is a big coil in my stomach trying to uncoil, it makes me want to growl at everyone. I'm very snappy and thinking of selling them BOTH!

March 31ˢᵗ
Decorated Steve's birthday cake. A big crocodile, with big teeth.... Bills idea.

April

April 1ˢᵗ
HAPPY BIRTHDAY AUNTIE YVONNE.
Lovings last night it seemed to release a huge pain. It came from deep inside like a huge wave.
I cried loud, ugly tears. My brain was shouting, it's over; it's over, no more nasty chemotherapy.
The relief left me completely drained and empty.
I held on to Steve and he cuddled me. Holding me close. After the tears had gone I looked at him. He was smiling. At that moment I felt that I had never been loved so much before in my life.
Today is the last day of the last week of having no immune system. I will never have to 'not' go in public places for a week ever again.
I've had a nasty headache all day, have resorted to taking a tablet.

April 2ⁿᵈ
My hands have gone all dry again, even though I am still taking the tablets.
Pope John Paul II died tonight.

April 3ʳᵈ
Had a birthday lunch for Steve. Mum and Dad came. Lucy was also down for the weekend.
Got a bit flustered, I feel as if I am panicking, I start to shake and seem not to have the confidence that I used to have. I don't know why. I had a few tears. I am having trouble concentrating, I think that my mind in occupied unconsciously with the radiotherapy treatments that are going to start soon. I wonder what it will be like. Chemotherapy

wasn't really that bad. I got away quite lightly seeing as there were lots of horrible side-effects and I didn't seem to get them too bad really, in my way of thinking that means that I am going to cop it with the side-effects of the radiotherapy.

April 4th

The inside of the elbow on the arm that I had chemotherapy given really hurts. It hurts when I stretch up and I have noticed that I have got no veins on that hand or arm. You know when you get hot or when you have your arm hanging down by the side of you you can see the veins? Well, I haven't got any, they have gone away, disappeared, vanished! My hand and arm are completely smooth, the other arm and hand are veiny, it's just the left one that isn't.

Went into town with the children. Bill fell over outside HMV, he landed with his hand on some broken glass. The manager in the shop was very kind and helped patch him up.

Lucy passed her driving test at 7:30 this morning.

I'm so pleased for her, Steve said her being on the road is going to make him completely grey through worry.

April 5th

HAPPY BIRTHDAY STEVE!

I am so tired today; I was tired when I woke up this morning. My whole self is tired. It's like someone has sucked out all my energy.

The children were no different than any other day, but today it was as if they were the noisiest, most horrible, demanding children in the whole world.

If I had thought about it or had the nerve, I would have got in the car and driven away......

No, I wouldn't, I haven't got the energy.

The health visitor came to see me at lunch time. We chatted and I told her that I wasn't coping very well. She gave me one of her looks and asked 'what I did I expect under the circumstances?' and that she thought that I was doing a 'marvellous job'.

I am not doing my exercises everyday now. Now I only do them when my arms feel a bit stiff. I still can't get used to seeing my 'boobs' moving and squashing as I move my arms. Sometimes it fascinates me, other times it just looks gross.

Weighed....9st 11lbs.

When I feel as low as I think that I can go I take all my clothes of and stand in front of the mirror and look at what cancer has turned me into.

My head is bald, my cheeks are hollow. I have huge scars that slash across my chest. I have two bowl shaped mounds where my breasts were, my ribs stick out and have 'bolts' on the sides. I have no body hair. I look like an alien. I feel repulsion when I look at myself. But then I pull a funny face and do a silly dance. I smile to myself. At least I am alive!

P.s. I only do this when I am on my own. Never with an audience. That would be so embarrasing.

April 6th

My first appointment at the Churchill Hospital in Oxford.

Dad and I left with loads of time to spare. We hit a little bit of traffic but got there in time.

We had to go up the stairs and along to the end of the corridor. We went into the waiting room and showed the receptionist our letter. She showed us where to wait. A nurse came and spoke to us after a while and said that they were running late and would we like to go to the canteen and have a drink and come back in about half an hour.

We went to the canteen and had a cheese roll and a cup of tea. When we got back we were seen straight away.

We went into a room that had a chair similar to the ones in the dentist. I was asked my name, date of birth and address.

They then asked me to take my top off, that was when Dad left the room.

I had to sit leaning back with my knees bent; my arms and hands were put into some cuffs that were above my head. Either side of me there were screens that showed my name and lots of numbers. They lowered a machine down and the lights were dimmed. Red lasers shone across me and made a grid, a white one also came across and made the image of a ruler on me. The radiographer made notes and recorded numbers, she drew a line down the middle of my breast bone, a mark where my nipple would have been on my right breast and several on my right side under my armpit and on my ribs.

They said that they needed to take an x-ray to make sure that the radiotherapy would just skim my lungs.

They were pleased with their calculations; my oncologist came in the room and double-checked everything.

The last thing that they did was make the marks they had drawn permanent and did this by getting a pot of ink and then stabbing me with a needle to leave a black spot. The one in the middle of my breastbone looks like a large black-head!

When they showed us out they pointed out the room that I would be having my treatments in.

Dad said our goodbyes and we left for home. I fell asleep in the car. I'm so tired, went to bed at 8 o'clock. Totally knackered.

April 7th

Feel a bit better this morning; don't know how long it will last.

My hair seems to be coming out? Went to the theatre this evening to see a Lonnie Donagan show. Its the first time out since my operation. Auntie Jill babysat, I was so excited that I nearly went out without a scarf, not quite brave enough yet.

I had a lovely time. Thinking about it, nobody seemed to look at me and I didn't think about anything apart from having a good time.

April 8th

Rotten day. Raining.

Kids bored, me bored. Hair still coming out..

Took the children to 'Space Adventure'.

They had a wonderful time, I had a hot chocolate.

Pope John Paul II funeral.

April 9th

Woke up tired again.

Kids all having a go at each other as I was putting the washing in the machine it all got too much and I cried. I can't cope. I seem to have too much to do all at the same time; even the thought of going shopping fills me with dread.

I get in the bath in the morning and have trouble finding the energy to move or get out. All I want to do is lay down and sleep, but I know that being a mum with four young children at home makes that an impossibility. So life carries on as normal!

Auntie Jill looked after Fred and I took Jake, Molly and Bill to the cinema. It was Bills first time, he was fascinated with the 'huge television'!

Prince Charles and Camilla got married today, I watched it on the television. Bit different to his last one, but he looked happier.

April 10^{*th*}

Weary.

That word fits exactly how I feel, I am weary.

Weary of being a mum. Weary of having cancer.

Weary of all the treatments. Weary of life?...No, because I know it is not going to last. Sunshine and warm weather would help. Having enough hair so that I didn't have to wear a scarf would help even more.

April 11^{*th*}

Sunshine! Woke up this morning to beautiful sunshine. My day started with a huge smile.

Jake and Molly are at school, Bill is at nursery.

This afternoon I had my scan. I left the children with our Auntie Jill. I took a book with me, secretly hoping to be kept waiting so that I could finish it. But, as soon as I sat down I was called in.

I was asked to loosen my trousers and pull my top up. A lovely smiley lady came in. She said that she was going to scan my womb and ovaries. As she was scanning she talked me through what she could see. My ovaries were fine and so was my womb.

She told me that my period would be in the next week because, she said pointing to the screen if I had just had one my womb would be showing up much whiter.

She said that while we were there that she would also check my liver, gall bladder and the bits in- between.

She asked me to lie on my side and she checked my kidneys and my spleen.

Everything was fine and exactly how it should be. She then said that to be completely sure that she would scan me from the inside. She asked me to go to the toilet and have a wee while she changed some of the bits of equipment around on the couch.

I took off my trousers and pants; I sat on the end of the couch. She asked me to lay back and place my legs up in some rests.

She used a scanner that looked like a fluorescent light tube. We saw my ovaries and womb from a different angle and she said that it confirmed that everything was as it should be. She said that she would write in her report that there were no abnormalities. As I was getting dressed I thanked her very much.

I asked her if these were the only parts of the body she scanned, meaning the lower parts of ladies, as I told her that Steve was coming in on Thursday.

She said that she scanned everything except scrotum's, I said that wasn't where his problem was, it was his leg. I laughed, it made me smile for the rest of the day.

I came out of the hospital back into sunshine, feeling relieved that there was nothing wrong. Maybe I had pulled a muscle and because I still carry the children it hasn't had a chance to heal? As I am writing this, I have just thought, I was not worried, or at all concerned about the scan today. All the others I have had a fear that they would find something wrong, but this one I just went to, without a second thought......weird?

April 12th

Woke up feeling more positive today. Cleaned the kitchen, re-oiled the beechwood counters.

Bill used the pedals on his trike. The sun shone. The birds sang. The trees are full of blossom and turning a beautiful fresh green with new leaves.

Steve and Jake went to speedway tonight.

April 13th

HAPPY BIRTHDAY AUNTIE SYLVIA.
Bill, Jake and Molly went to school.

Fred and I went to Coate Water. We fed the ducks and had a lovely walk. It revived me and made me feel alive. Came back and had a cup of tea.

Smiling today.

April 14th

Bill has got conjunctivitis.

Steve got up late this morning and as he got in the van he split his tea on his leg. He didn't go to work today....not in a very good mood. I improved this by taking him with me to buy a new hoover! In the afternoon he had his scan on his leg, it was inconclusive and in his colourful way of explaining things, a waste of time.

April 15th

Fred has got conjunctivitis.

Lucy drove down, for the first time.

It's very cold today.

April 16th

Thank you boys I also have conjunctivitis.

Molly is sleeping over at a friends house tonight. Went to Boots with her and got loads of girly things for them to do; face masks, make-up and nail varnish.

April 18th

Bill worried his teachers at nursery today. He decided to hide when it was time to come in from play and they couldn't find him.

They found him giggling round the corner!

April 19th

HAPPY BIRTHDAY DARREN.

April 21st

Started my period today.

April 22nd

Molly had another football match.

April 23rd

Today I woke up feeling fantastic, but after I had had a bath I felt really sad. I was sad but also cross inside. I couldn't be bothered to talk or answer anyone.

Poor Steve got the brunt of it again. I didn't look at him. As far as I was concerned he could just go away. All I wanted to do was cry. Every time someone spoke to me I cried. This mood lasted 'til the afternoon.

I went upstairs and all I could hear was, "Mum, Mum, Mum," followed by loads of questions. I went into our bedroom and sat on the floor behind the bed and cried and cried. Steve came in and held me. We stayed like that for what seemed like ages. Once the tears had gone I got up and felt completely normal and calm.

I don't understand why it happens, but once the big tears come out, it's all over.

Molly went to a friends party, 12 till 2.

Steve and I took Bill to see 'Bananas in Pyjamas' at the theatre. It was brilliant......... if you were 2!

Jake slept over at a friends.

April 25th

Got a letter, Bill has got a place at pre-school, he starts in September.

April 26th

John has gone on holiday to Spain with loads of friends.

Went to watch Molly play in the school netball tournament.

The supermarket has stopped doing my teabags so I have gone on to a new one; Dr Stuarts Echinacea Plus, it is quite nice, they also say that echinacea is good for the immune system, so it might give it a boost..

I'm not superstitious by any means but I do wear my knickers with buttercups on every time I have an appointment with the oncologists or surgeons or doctors. I always wear them when I had my chemotherapy treatments. As I say, I"m not superstitious at all!

Chapter 6

April 27ᵗʰ

My Mum came down to stay for a week.

Today is the first one of the radiotherapy appointments.

I have decided that I am not going to wear my head scarf because the hospital is a cancer one, so, everyone that goes there is in a similar situation to me and no one will take any notice of my head, anyway I reckon that it doesn't look that bad.

We left with a good hour to get there and made it just in time. We went inside and booked in.

Mum stayed with Bill and Fred in the main waiting room and I went up and waited outside the room that I would be having my treatment in.

I got chatting to two ladies while I was waiting. One lady was having treatment on her breasts, like me and the other lady was having treatment on her jaw because it had been found in her salivary glands. Her name is Joy.

It was so nice being able to chat to people in the same boat as me and swap 'horror' stories about chemotherapy and losing hair and being sick and feeling sick.

It was like a breath of fresh air talking and listening to people going through the same as me.

It doesn't matter how understanding other people are when you tell them what you are going through, it is not the same as discussing it with someone who is going through it as well.

After what seemed like ages I was called in.

The room was huge. Its walls were covered with wooden panelling. There was a machine in the middle of the room with a bed incorporated into it. It had rests for your arms to be placed above your head and a rest so that your knees stayed bent.

In the room with me was a radiologist and a nurse. They talked me through what they were going to do. The machine had a large disc with a lens in the middle which went at the side of me and there was a screen up on the wall which showed lots of numbers to do with the degrees of the bed and other angles.

They measured me and set the machine up then left the room with me in it, spread eagled on the bed. I felt like a sacrifice, very vulnerable.

(It was a good job that I checked my spelling as I originally wrote venerable, not vulnerable and venerable means; accorded great respect because of age, wisdom, or character; a title given to an archdeacon, not quite the same thing is it?)

The machine beeped thirty-five times, wurred and then stopped. The nurse and radiologist came back in and the machine was moved so that it was pointing to the other side of me. Again they left the room and the machine beeped thirty-five times, wurred and then stopped.

When they returned they said that I could move my arms and sit up. "All done." They said.

I thanked them and said I would see them in the morning and off I went. We went home, I felt fine. But, by half past six I was sound asleep.

It had rained all day, but I went a whole day with my head uncovered and I didn't feel self conscious at all. I've done it once so there is no going back. The head scarfs are banished to the bottom drawer until they become fashionable. 24 treatments to go.

April 28ᵗʰ

The same as yesterday but I fell asleep in the car on the way home.

Molly played football for her school team. They lost 2-0. Jake and Steve went to speedway.

Johns flight is delayed, he is coming home tomorrow.

23 treatments to go.

April 29ᵗʰ

Felt sick this morning, but was o.k. Radiotherapy went fine. Breast is a bit sore, still putting on E45.

22 treatments to go.

May

May 1ˢᵗ

This morning Bill decided to fill the toilet bowl up with paper and then flushed it. It overflowed and flooded the bathroom and came through the kitchen ceiling.

We had to buy a new carpet for the bathroom, the old one couldn't be saved.. Steve had to dismantle the toilet to unblock it. Not a good start to the day.

Nice roast pork dinner, though.

May 3ʳᵈ

Today is my only early appointment, 9:30am.

All the others are at 11:12 or later.

We got the children ready and had to leave the house at 8 o'clock because we would hit the rush hour.

When we got to the hospital there was a notice saying that one of the machines had broken down so they were alternating patients from both machines to one. We had to wait quite a while and we need not have rushed to get there, never mind. Went to the shops on the way home and we were back and all finished by 1 o'clock.

At home there was a letter asking me to go for an interview. I had forgotten about the job because I had applied for it last September, interview date 17ᵗʰ May.

21 treatments to go.

May 4ᵗʰ

My Mum went home today.

May 5ᵗʰ

General Election, Blair got in again. Bugger!

May 6ᵗʰ

Dad took me to the hospital today. In the toilets I was accosted by a lady. "I know you." she said. She told me that we had had chemotherapy with each other at the Great Western Hospital.

I felt awful because I didn't recognise her.

We talked together as we walked up to the waiting room and didn't stop talking until we were both called in.

It was refreshing talking to her; she was having the same treatment, for the same illness.

She had also had the same type of chemotherapy as me. It made me feel a bit better knowing someone else had experienced it at the same time as me. It was a real boost seeing her, as she looked healthy and happy.

It made how I felt seem normal. (Also she had put on a stone with her treatment and I had only put on 13lbs!)

May 7ᵗʰ

Sunshine. Lovely warm sunshine. Felt much more positive again today. Also feeling a bit ashamed that I have been wallowing in a lot of self-pity.

Washed the windows inside and out. Fish and chips for tea.

May 8ᵗʰ

9st today! Feeling even happier.

My moods are totally erratic. The not only swing from day to day, but from hour to hour.

May 9ᵗʰ

Steve had the day off today so he took me to the hospital.

He came in while they set me up and they talked him through what they are doing.

Fell asleep on the way home. Very tired today.

Jake started his sats today and Molly started her year 5 exams.

May 10ᵗʰ

Today the nurse said that I smelt nice.

Brought Fred some new shoes, size 6 1/2H!

17 treatments to go.

May 11ᵗʰ

Bill is at school today so I thought that I would drive myself.

Tonight I am so tired that it made me cry. Steve told me that would happen. He asked me not to drive myself again.

I have pin and needles in my left leg, from the knee down and in my left arm from the elbow down.

My hair is growing nicely. I have the most hair of all the people in the waiting room. I am the only one without a hat! Had to shave my armpits again.

Health visitor came round again for a good old natter.

16 treatments to go.

May 12ᵗʰ

As I laid down to have my treatment my left leg felt very strange, pins and needles, numbness and cold all at the same time. It also felt like my hip was being pulled. Once I had moved it felt better again.

When I got home I picked Fred up and my lower back gave me a right old jolt. I couldn't right myself properly. It didn't get any better when I changed my position so I rang the chiropractor and managed to get an appointment for that afternoon. She worked her magic once again.

May 13ᵗʰ

The journey to the hospital goes all through the countryside on all the back roads. It is really pretty, all there is, is fields and woodland.

There is one bit of woodland that has got a house hidden in it that looks just like 'Snow Whites'. You can imagine the dwarfs and animals all being quite at home there.

Also there is a hill that is covered with huge trees. Hidden in between them is a tower that I am sure still holds Rapunsel as a prisoner!.

May 14ᵗʰ

This morning after my bath I caught a glimpse of myself in the mirror and noticed that I have a red square of skin that covers my right breast.

It also reassured me that the radiotherapy was actually doing something, I had started to think that it was just a placebo!

I'm quite happy because it covers half of my armpit and that is where the lymph nodes were taken from. I remember asking the oncologist if they were going to do radiotherapy on my armpit and he had said no because it can sometimes cause the arm swell. I thought that it was a bit strange because they were doing radiotherapy on the breast as a safety measure as backup for the chemotherapy , yet if cancerous cells were found in the armpit they should be taking the same measures, but they weren't. But by looking at the redness, indirectly they were.

May 15th

This illness had made me notice nature more than I have before. The bird's songs are louder and more beautiful, the leaves on the trees are such a vibrant kaleidoscope of greens.

Flowers seem more delicate and intricate the breeze has a magic of its own that I never noticed before. You take a deep breath and thank God that you are alive.

May 16th

I think that it would hurt much more if I had feeling in my breasts, but, I only have feeling around the breasts not on them. My right breast is really sore today, especially just above it. It's true that is does feel like bad sun burn. The nurse advised me to put my E45 in the fridge so that it is cold when I put it on. It didn't feel any better, just cold and it makes me flinch.

13 treatments to go.

May 17th

Front page news this morning. Kylie Minogue has breast cancer. On the radio all day, everyone who has had cancer was ringing up and giving advice to her. They also played one of her songs; 'I should be so lucky.'......Not one of the best choices. At the beginning, the last thing you want to be told is how well everyone else coped through the illness......well that is how I felt anyway. It's like being told how fantastic pregnancy is, when you have got morning sickness all day. My period has started.

Had a job interview this afternoon. Congratulations me! I got the job. I start as soon as the C.R.B. checks come back. I am so happy, I came out of the interview and the sun was shinning and I felt so clever. My short hair didn't put them off me. To them I looked normal. What a boost. I am no longer in the 'cancer patient' category by means of looks any more. I keep smiling. I am so happy.

Molly had a football match against Penhill. Her team lost 11-0!!! She was still smiling though.

May 18ᵗʰ

Happy Anniversary Us.

Steve had the day off, so he took me to the hospital. Still smiling. Still so happy. Sun is still shinning. If I had to describe myself I would say that I am very lucky.

11 treatments to go.

May 19ᵗʰ

Some of the road that we travel on to the hospital runs parallel with the railway. Today Dad and I were caught in a bit of traffic, when a train went passed. I pointed out the train to Bill and Fred and then laughed because, when Jake and Molly had been about the same age, my Mum and I had been driving back from Bournmouth. We had been stuck in traffic along a piece of road with a train line running along side it.

I had pointed out a train to them and, not looking at the road had driven into the back of the car in front of me. When I explained to that driver that I had been showing the children the train and that I was sorry that I had hit his car, he hadn't seemed very impressed. No damaged was caused. We weren't going fast enough.

May 20ᵗʰ

Bill and Fred are fantastic!

Every day they sit in the car for an hour there and an hour back, good as gold. They walk into the hospital as if it is second nature, saying 'hello' to everyone.

They go in there and chat to the huge fish in the fish tank in the waiting room. Then go into the corner and play with the toys while I am inside having my treatment. Fred is just as good on his own on a

Monday and Wednesday, when he comes on his own with us because Bill has school and is picked up by Auntie Jill, who gives him his lunch.

May 21ˢᵗ

After lovings tonight I felt very scared. A huge fear came over me. Lovings makes me feel so alive, every inch of me. Then when it is over I hope that it has not been the last time. I know that it isn't, but it could have been. So maybe I cry because I am grateful to be alive or maybe its because I also realize how close I came to death.

If I hadn't gone to the doctor when I did and if it hadn't been diagnosed then, yes, I could be dead now, and the bonding we have when loving makes me feel ecstatic and frightened all at the same time. It heightens all my emotions.

May 22ⁿᵈ

Saw myself in the mirror again and my square is not just red, but bright red, lobster red! I look very strange.. It has started to itch in the top left hand corner. Got a letter from the 'social' apparently having cancer and all the treatments that go with it does not disable or incapacitate you enough not to work! Therefore I am not entitled to any benefit. Maybe next time I will just pull a muscle in my back! They did say that they would pay my stamp though.

May 23ʳᵈ

Steve is taking me to the hospital today, tomorrow and Wednesday.

Bill was sick again this morning, that makes three days.

Got an appointment at the doctors, he told me that Bill has got a virus. That is what they always call it.

May 24ᵗʰ

I have noticed that when I walk up the stairs, I get out of breath easily. I have to stand and wait to get my breath back, just like an old lady. On the telephone tonight I told Mum that it was happening and she said that she had felt the same way as well. It always makes me feel better when someone else has had the same thing. Then you know that it isn't serious.

Jake, Molly and Bill have broken up for half term.

7 treatments to go.

May 26ᵗʰ

My Mum has come down to help with the driving for the last week.

I asked the radiographer yesterday if Jake could come in with me and see what was done.

Jake and I left the others in the waiting room and we went up and sat outside the treatment room.

We were soon called in and Jake was talked through what they did to me. He came out disillusioned with what I was having done.

I think he thought 'Is that it? Is that what all the fuss is about?'..... I hope he never finds out.

On the way out we went to the clinical genetics department and gave in a form that I had filled out with all the family history. It showed who had died of what, mainly cancer, to find out if there is a genetic link to who gets which cancer.

I did it to see if Molly was at a high risk of developing breast cancer or whether Mum and I were just dealt bad luck.

May 27ᵗʰ

On the way to the hospital today our breath was taken away by the sight of the fields, they were full to bursting with the most beautiful red poppies that we had ever seen.

If we had had the time we could had just stared for hours...... Wow.

May 29ᵗʰ

Today we had a party for Lucy's birthday. Mum and Dad came over. Altogether there were eleven of us. We had a lovely day. It was brilliant fun! Everything was pink!

May 31st

HAPPY BIRTHDAY LUCY!

Three days left! I can't believe it. Now it seems to have gone so quickly. The year is going so fast, it is June tomorrow, half way through the year already!

Joy, who I see every day and have a chat to is having her last treatment today. She has given me a card, on which she has written instructions on the front that I am not allowed to open it until I finish my course of treatment.

I am so tired today. So sleepy.

I am so glad that my Mum is here.

June

June 1st

One day to go! Everyone keeps reminding me.

Molly is going to speedway with Steve tomorrow night for the first time, she is ever so excited.

June 2nd

Last radiotherapy treatment.

When I went into the room and ALL the radiologists and nurses came in as well.

(Good job I don't get embarrassed easily.) It was nice to know that they liked me. I was given a cuddle as I left and given loads of good wishes. I blubbed. It was an 'Oh, my God, this nightmare is finally over and I have got through it,' kind of blub.

The relief was almost physical. I got back to the waiting room where Mum and the children were waiting. Mum took one look at me and gave me a huge hug. I gave a form into the receptionist and was told an appointment would be made with the oncologist in about four weeks time at the Great Western Hospital for a check up. We left and said goodbye to the Churchill Hospital, Oxford.

Chapter 7

―――◈―――

When I got home I opened the card that Joy had given me. Inside it wished me all the best for a healthy future and it also had two passages from the bible for me to look up.

They were; Jeremiah 29 v11-13 and Isaiah 40 v28-30.

"For I know the plans I have for you" declares the Lord, "plans to prosper you and not to harm you, plans to give you hope and a future. Then you will call upon me and come and pray to me, and I will listen to you. You will seek me and find me when you seek me with all your heart."

and,

Do you not know? Have you not heard? The Lord is the everlasting God, the Creator of the ends of the earth. He will not grow tired or weary, and his understanding no-one can fathom.

He gives strength to the weary and increases the power of the weak. Even youths grow tired and weary, and the young men stumble and fall:

When I first read them I didn't understand why she had chosen these passages, but when I read them a couple of weeks later they made more sense to me. You go through hardship or illness and while you are there you cannot see an end to it, but once it is over you return to your old self and energy it just becomes part of your past, your history that makes you you, and I think that you become a better person for the bad things in life. It makes you whole and complete rather than shallow and self obsessed. You see the courage and determination in the every day people that you would normally pass by without a second glance.

I'm not saying that if you get cancer or any other illness that you should turn to God or start going to church and become a 'bible basher', but everything happens for a reason and that reason is not always clear.

In the bible you can read stories or parables that you can relate to certain characters that you find are in your own life.

People read horoscopes in the daily papers but reading a verse or chapter from the bible would be just the same.

When I look at myself in the mirror I am glad that I decided to have a double mastectomy because both breasts look the same. I don't have one that looks like the old me and one that has been disfigured, I am just me. I may not have nipples but that doesn't matter because there is nothing to compare them with.

When I have got clothes on, I have a figure that I am sure some women would envy. I am not angry or resentful for having to have the surgery. I am not angry or resentful for having cancer. I am just me. Tania Bond, wife, mother, daughter, granddaughter, sister, auntie, niece, cousin, friend, neighbour and the woman who lives down the road, who experienced something in her life that she chose to write a book about.

I was also very lucky. Steve and I managed to keep every day life as normal as we could for the children. The side-effects didn't stop the mundane day to day routine from being disrupted too much. I don't think that we fooled anyone into thinking that there was nothing wrong, but we managed to protect the children from the worry and emotional pain that this disease brings with it.

I am not saying that we have all come out of this unscathed, but keeping life as normal as you can does seem to dampen the seriousness of the disease and make it a molehill rather than a mountain to climb.

What have I got out of having breast cancer?

1) After a bath when you wrap a towel round you, it doesn't fall down because when you have a double mastectomy they don't move or change shape.

2) You can go out in the cold and not look it. No nipples.

3) You don't have to wear a bra, no ugly straps to spoil an outfit.

4) They don't bounce around when you run.

5) You are a hit of Halloween with the children because you have real 'bolts' coming out of your sides.

6) You can choose what size they are made. Free boob job.

7) You get to see what you look like bald.

8) You realize how much and how many people love and care for you.

9) You realise how precious and fragile life is. Life is truly a unique gift to be treasured.

Thank You Everyone. For everything. Love from Tan.

x x x

P.s July 7th My first appointment with the oncologist after all the treatment.

"Mrs. Bond, I am pleased to say, at this moment in time there is no cancer in your body."

August 10th 2005.

Chapter 8

——◆——

I wasn't going to write any more of this diary but certain things happen in day to day life that I wanted to tell someone.

Like the time that I was shopping. I was leaning over the trolley to unload my shopping and I caught the eye of a man. He smiled at me, then I noticed that his eyes wandered to my top that I hadn't noticed was gaping open.

His look went from being one of smiles to one of disgust.

When I looked at my cleavage I saw what he had seen.

I saw a mutilated and disfigured pair of breasts. Actually they looked nothing like a pair of breasts. The way that they had been rebuilt meant that the implants were put behind the muscles, so every time I used my arms, the muscles were contracting causing the breasts to change shape.

It hasn't stopped me wearing tops that are a bit revealing, but when I catch sight of myself for example, doing the gardening it makes me a bit self conscious.

August

August 12th

Today we put our house on the market. It is too small with all the children and also the area has gone to the dogs, rubbish everywhere, youths hanging around and being intimidating, generally society is regressing.

August 14th

My hair is about an inch long, maybe longer,I have started gelling it and giving it an 'unkept' look.

We spent the day at Robert and Margo's down at Hayling Island. They laid on a BBQ and we all had a lovely time. All the family were there and it was a wonderful day.

August 15th

This morning I noticed that there was some blood on my pillow when I woke up. I couldn't think where it had come from and I assumed that it was from Steve and that he had cut himself shaving last night.

August 16th

There was blood on my pillow again this morning, I felt the back of my neck and there was a scab on the mole at the back of my neck near my left ear. I looked at it in the mirror.

My heart sank. Had it come back, but this time in my skin? I rang the doctors and made an appointment. The earliest they can fit me in is Monday at 8;40. I am getting myself in a right old pickle. I spend most of the day with my hand touching the mole and looking in the mirror to see if it is better. I keep checking it. Maybe I had made a mistake and that it wasn't really bleeding after all?

August 18th

Made and decorated Molly cake. Bill customized it by rubbing his hands all over it. Thank you very much Bill.

August 19th

HAPPY BIRTHDAY MOLLY!

Since I have finished having my treatments I feel a strange mix of emotions. All the time that I was having scans and x-rays before my operations the breast care nurses were telephoning and keeping a check on me to make sure that I was alright, then when I was having chemotherapy, people were concerned for my well being including the oncologists. The radiotherapy involved someone being with me every day, either Dad, Steve or my Mum and now that the treatments are all over I am returned to the background, not that I want the treatments to continue or be ill and have to be monitored by specialists but it was quite nice just for a while being the centre of attention and my days feel empty now that I am out of the 'limelight'.

I seem to have too much time in the day because instead of fitting all the housework and shopping ect around the treatments I have all day to do it.

August 20th

Lady came round to view the house today. She fell in love with it. She asked to come back tomorrow with her husband.

August 21st

He seems impressed as well. They are going to see the estate agent in the morning.

August 22nd

I have my doctors appointment this morning. I told her about the mole on the back of my neck. She checked it. She told me that it was fine and that I had just caught it on something. I told her the panic that I had got myself into and I asked her if you ever stop thinking that everything is the cancer and that it has come back?.

She said no, you don't but that eventually you know that every ache, pain, feeling and sensation that is not normal does not mean that it has returned. She said that I will never feel the way that I did before the cancer. She said that I will never be as fit or as healthy as I was and that I will always have aches and pains that are new to me. She said that I will always think that it has returned but there is always someone, either at the hospital or at the doctors to put my mind at rest. She said that eventually I will be able to live my life as well as I did but that it takes a long time to learn to live with the shadow of cancer that follows you every day.

She also told me that she was leaving the practice.

It caused me to panic slightly. She had been with me from when I had first been diagnosed and knew how I felt and could offer genuine sympathy when I needed it.

TODAY WE SOLD OUR HOUSE!!!!!!!

August 23rd

Molly has gone to Nan's for a couple of days, when she is there she is totally spoilt and goes horse riding. She went with Steve this morning when he went to work. Poor Molly will be so tired. They left at 6 o'clock.

Jake didn't go to school today because he has been sick. Molly said that he had been eating blackberries.....Serves him right. We have told him so many times not to.

August 24th

Jake seems a bit better today. He has stopped being sick but he still has an upset tummy.

Bill and I went into town to pick up some house details.

We need a new home!

August 25th

Jake has started being sick again and is having trouble going to the toilet.

I called the doctor and asked if she could come and do a home visit. She said that she would be here at lunchtime. She says that he has got a urine infection and has prescribed some antibiotics for him.

This evening Steve and I went to look at some houses......Yuck, apart from one which is a bit out of out price range.

August 26th

Early this morning I rang the out of hours doctor because Jake is in so much pain. They were not at all helpful. They said that the surgery would be open soon and to call them! Jake seemed better later on, but by lunchtime he was confined to the bathroom being violently sick. I called the doctors again and she came straight round. Jake was lying on the bathroom floor unable to move because of the pain in his stomach. The doctor felt his stomach and said that he had a suspected appendicitis. She rang the hospital to say that he was on his way. She asked if I could get him to the hospital. I telephoned several of our friends but no one was at home and there was no way that I would be able to move him on my own so we called an ambulance.

In the mean time I rang Mum and Dad, they came over with Molly.

Auntie Jill came in from next door to look after Bill and Fred. The ambulance arrived to take Jake and I to the hospital. When we got to the hospital we had to wait a little while until a cubicle was empty. We were put in cubicle 19. Jakes birthday is the 19th. The house that we had seen and liked very much was number 19. An omen maybe?

Jake was seen by a nurse and had his temperature taken. It was very high. They gave him some medicine to take his temperature down and some more for the pain. He was admitted to the children's ward. He was seen by a surgeon and then the head surgeon. Steve arrived and we were told that they were going to operate. They put some magic cream on his hands and arms so that they it wouldn't hurt too much when they put the cannula in.

Steve went home and I stayed until they took him down to the operating theatre .He looked so tiny on the trolley as they put him to sleep. It was 8 o'clock and they said the operation should take about half an hour and then he would be in resus for another another half an hour. I told them I would be back at quarter to nine after I had put Bill and Fred to bed and told everyone what was happening. I got back at quarter to nine and went to the children's ward. The nurses said that there was no news yet but as soon as there was I could go down the the theater and bring him up with them. I went into the parents room and made myself a cup of tea. I kept looking at the clock. It got to half past nine. I started to worry. It had been too long. I went and spoke to the nurses. They said that they had had no news but would ring down for me. They were told that Jake was in resus. At ten o'clock the nurses came in to the parents room. Jake had woken up. I went down with one of the nurses. It was so quiet in the hospital with everyone asleep and no visitors.

In the area where all the theatres are it was deserted as well.

We stood not knowing quite where to go until we spotted someone and they directed us in the right direction. We opened a set of double doors and behind some curtains was Jake looking very sleepy. He opened his eyes. "Hello, Mum." he said giving me a huge smile. I went over and gave him a big cuddle. He started fiddling with his gown.

He was trying to show me his scar, but instead was showing everyone a whole lot more as the gown was the only thing he had on!

The nurse that was looking after him said that he was a very polite and well mannered child and that it has been a pleasure to look after him.

She has written out a certificate that said he had been very brave having his operation.

As we left, Jake thanked everyone for looking after him and said that he would see them again tomorrow!

Back on the ward we settled him down and I gave him a kiss and cuddle and said that I would see him in the morning.

August 27ᵗʰ

Jake is a lot better today. (He couldn't of been any worse than yesterday lunchtime!)

The surgeon came round and said that Jake had been a very lucky young man. He said that his appendix had gone gangrenous and his abdomen had been full of puss. He said that they had been surprised at the size of Jakes appendix as it had been a lot larger than found in a normal child of his age. He said that they were going to put him on a large dose of antibiotics for two days just in case there was any infection there and he should be able to go home after that. I stayed with Jake for the morning and then went home. Steve went and saw him in the afternoon and I went back at teatime.

He was much better and let me get him up and give him a wash and change his clothes.

In the evening he was very quiet. He was on a drip and was being given morphine for the pain. He had had the cannula changed to the other arm and was feeling a bit sorry for himself.

I settled him down for the night and came home.

August 28ᵗʰ

Jakes ward is up several flights of stairs and I always take them rather than using the lift, but I am finding that I am getting even more out of breath. It is making my chest feel very tight. I also end up coughing and causing a rattle in my throat. I think that I am becoming a hypochondriac, either that or I am dying!

Today they gave Jake some food, it made him sick all night!

Went to look at the house that was out of our price range again, but this time we went inside. We have found our dream house.

August 29th

Jake was sick again this morning so they have put him back on a drip, without food.

Steve had the day of work so we went up together to see him.

This evening I had an appointment with the surgeon to see how I am getting on. Steve came with me. He checked me over and asked me some questions. I told him that I had a chesty cough and that I was still very breathless. I said that I was still getting nausea and also that I always seemed tired. He sat and listened. He said that it was still early days and that it would take the body a long time to recover because essentially my system had been poisoned and it needed time to get better. He checked my implants and listened to my chest and back. He said that he would order a chest x-ray just to make sure that there was nothing sinister going on. I said that the implants were becoming uncomfortable and asked when they could be removed and the proper ones could be put in. He said that because it hadn't been long since I had had all the treatments he would rather wait until he saw me in February.

We left and went back downstairs to Jake. I settled him down for the night and we came home.

John had been looking after Bill, Fred and Molly so after a cup of tea Steve took him home.

August 30th

Had my chest x-ray this morning and them we went to see Jake.

The boys and Molly played outside, we took Jake out in a wheelchair.

Steve was late home.

We had thunder and lightening, heavy rain and poor Steve got a puncture in the works van with no tools or spare so had to wait for the AA.

Not a happy man when he got home.

August 31st

Today they took Jake off his drip and he had some macaroni cheese for his lunch.

He seems a bit happier.

Got a speeding ticket. Sixty pounds. 3 Points.

Bugger!

September

September 1st

The hospital told us that Jake is coming home tomorrow. Our offer has been excepted on the house that we want. Very posh, five bedrooms, two bathrooms and three toilets!!!!

September 2nd ,

JAKE CAME HOME.

They gave his some antibiotics that he would finish on Sunday.

September 3rd

Dug up all the plants that I am taking to the new house. Got my driving license back with the addition of my new points.

Lucy is down for the weekend.

September 4th

Everybody is here today. Seems ages since it has been like this.

I have started getting dizzy spells, well its not quite like dizziness. It is like the feeling you get when you have been on a boat and once you are on dry land you find that you still have your sea legs. I have also got a stinking headache that I can't seem to shift.

I don't help myself as I have been reading the Caron Keating story in the Daily Mail. The amount of times Steve tells me not to read articles about cancer and how different people have coped and survived or died courageously. All it does is make you think and you end up feeling and thinking that you have the same symptoms that you are reading about. Definitely not self-help reading.

September 5th

Had an appointment at the doctors.

She said that I have Labrythitus and has given me some tablets.

Packed the kitchen ready to move. Lucy went home.

September 7th

Took all the mortgage stuff into the Abbey to get signed and stamped. Sent off. Jake had an appointment at the doctors.

She examined his stomach and telephoned the hospital. He is to be re-admitted. I telephoned Bills nursery and they are going to keep him there until 6 o'clock. Auntie Jill is going to have Fred and look after Molly when she comes home.

Jake is back on the children's ward. He is given an x-ray and a scan. He is put back onto a drip.

They have found an abscess in his abdomen about the size of a tennis ball. They may have to operate again.

September 8th

Mum and Dad have come down to take the boys home with them. What would I do without them?

Went to visit Jake. He seems better, it must be the antibiotics that they are giving him.

After school I took Molly in and we all played Monopoly.

Uncle Ron and Auntie Sylvia went to Canada for a wedding.

I cancelled Bills home visit for pre-school.

September 9th

Today Jake is in a lot of pain. They have started giving him morphine again.

He was sick all night.

It is the most horrible feeling in the world when your child is in pain and there is nothing that you can do except sit and wait as it it too painful for them to move or have a cuddle. I left and on the way home I cried.

My Mum and Ian are going away for the weekend for a wedding.

September 10ᵗʰ

This morning I went to see my healer. I felt the calmness wash over me as she worked.

Jake is better today. I washed him and changed his clothes. He is still on a drip so still no food.

September 11ᵗʰ

Went to see Jake this morning. He looks fantastic. He is allowed to eat today, so I am going to take up some lunch. Roast beef Sunday lunch. In the evening we went for a little walk up the corridor, well I did, he was in a wheelchair.

September 13ᵗʰ

JAKE CAME HOME...AGAIN!

This time he has come home with loads of different tablets and two types of antibiotics to last for two weeks.

September 14ᵗʰ

Today Jakes teacher came round with some work for him as he is not allowed to return to school for two weeks. At the beginning of the month he was supposed to start at Dorcan Technological College, but he hasn't got there yet.

Sent some documents to the solicitor, recorded delivery. Went to the art shop and got some bits and pieces for Jake to make a present for his granddads birthday.

Still going light headed and dizzy.

Started taking anti-sickness again.

September 15ᵗʰ

Boys coming home today. John coming home for tea. Feeling rotten.

September 17ᵗʰ

Went with Steve to the theatre. It was supposed to be comedy. I didn't think that they were funny.

I feel like I have to hold on to things in case I fall over!

September 19th

HAPPY BIRTHDAY DAD!

Jake has an appointment at the hospital for a scan. The abscess has gone away. No trace of it.

Molly has football practice 3 till 4.

September 20th

All the children are having their hairs cut ready for their school photo.

Feeling sick again, took some anti-sickness.

September 21st

Got Fred's birthday present.

Changed Jakes school uniform as it is too big for him. Sent mortgage stuff of to the solicitor.

September 22nd

Went to Mum and Dads. Dad has brought an open topped taxi. He took us up and down the yard. All the time you are in it, it makes you smile. You feel like the Cheshire Cat from Alice in Wonderland.

Got a phone call from the hospital saying that an appointment had been made for me to see the surgeon on Tuesday night....It could only be the results of the chest x-ray.

September 23rd

HAPPY BIRTHDAY AUNTIE EILEEN.

The children had their school photo this morning. It is all done posh now and you can see and have a copy of it immediately.

Today I have got myself in a right old pickle.

I am shaking, the dizziness and feeling of light headiness is getting awful.

I keep coughing and thinking that the cancer is in my lungs!! Then I think that it has gone into my brain!! I don't know what to do, I want a cuddle and to be told that I am fine. I can't ring Steve as he is working in Southampton and anyway he wouldn't appreciate the phone call. My mum lives too far away. Steve's mum would only get in a fluster and end up with a bad migraine, so I rang the hospital and asked for the oncology department. They listened and put me through to the breast cancer nurse. She listened and said that unfortunately there was no clinic that day but she would fit me in on the Monday. She suggested that I made an appointment to see my doctor that day and she would be in touch. I rang the doctors and got an emergency appointment. I told her what I was feeling. She listened and said that in her opinion I was suffering from anxiety. She said that Labrythitus can last for weeks on end and that the tablets can only alleviate the symptoms it produces and that the virus has to work it way out on its own.

She said that every time you have it it takes longer to clear itself up.

I asked if it will get any easier, thinking that everything is cancer and she said, no. I went home feeling a bit better, but not much. I hate cancer and everything that goes with it. The breast cancer nurse rang back and said that I had an appointment at 12 o'clock on Monday. I told her what the doctor had said and she said to still go along just to make sure.

September 24th

Today it is a year since I was diagnosed with cancer. What do you do. Do you celebrate?

It can't go unnoticed so....Its noticed.

Went to Coate Water with the boys this morning.

There were loads of leaves to kick all around.

Fred says Coate Water like a French man, Coate War-tur!

September 25th

Lazy Sunday. Auntie Eileen rang today. It was lovely to hear her voice and have a chat. It also made me feel guilty for not keeping in touch in other ways than birthdays, Easter and Christmas cards.

She said that she had been in hospital with a blood clot in her leg, we had a laugh as we discussed the surgical stockings that you have to wear and how attractive they were.

September 26th

This morning Jake had an appointment to have a scan done. He was told to drink loads, which in true Jake fashion he decided wasn't necessary so he had to have the scan done twice.

I had my appointment with the oncologist at 12 o'clock. She sat me down. I told her that I was frightened that it had come back, in my lungs and in my brain. I told her all the symptoms that I have been having. She did some tests on my reflexes, and some tests with my eyes and tested my muscles. She said that she agreed with my doctor that I was suffering from anxiety and Labrynthitus.

I wanted to find out the results of the chest x-ray that I had, so, I took a deep breath and asked her. I explained that I had been telephoned on Thursday night and been told that an extra appointment had been arranged.

I was brought up to always look at the person talking to me in their eyes as it was extremely rude not to give that person your full attention, but, it was so difficult because as she was talking my chest x-ray came up on the computer screen. She looked at it and used the mouse to magnify one bit of it. Gloom filled my stomach. She looked at me and smiled. "I can't see anything 'sinister'." she said. I breathed an enormous sigh of relief. I then asked her to explain what she could see and to tell me what the bit was that she had magnified. The bit she had magnified was the lymph nodes, everyone has them and mine were fine. The shadowy bit on the left was my heart. All fine no problems. I thanked her so very much and went home.

Jake had an appointment at 2;10pm with his consultant. They looked at the scans and were very pleased with the results and said that they would see him again in six weeks.

September 27th

This evening Steve and I went to the hospital. I was optimistic as I knew that there wasn't anything wrong with my x-ray so maybe they had changed their minds and were going to operate early? We sat down with the surgeon. He looked as bemused as us. He had no idea why we had been called in either. He said that he was sorry and that he would telephone tomorrow with an explanation as to why we had been called in.

September 28th

HAPPY BIRTHDAY AUNTIE JILL.

Fred had his appointment at the foot clinic. They are pleased with his progress and do not want to see him again.

We gave Auntie Jill her present. She was ever so pleased. It was a hard back edition of her favourite novel.

The surgeon rang and said that he could offer no explanation as to why we were called in and could only apologise.

The dizziness and light headiness seems to be going away. Maybe the doctors were right. Anxiety. I must learn to slow down and let other people help. I don't have to do everything myself.

I looked up Anxious in the dictionary and this is what is said;

1) experiencing worry, nervousness, or unease.

2) very eager and concerned to do something or for something to happen.

It also said that it originates from the Latin word anxius (from angere 'to choke').

Which I metaphorically understand, in my way of thinking, that I am choking my spirit and stopping myself living life to the full. Writing this book is saving me hundreds of pounds that I would have spent seeing a psychologists. I am self diagnosing myself!

October

October 1st

HAPPY BIRTHDAY FRED!

This birthday was a lot better than last year as I was having a liver scan.

This year we have balloons, cake, streamers and fun!

October 2ⁿᵈ

Jake and Molly have found a new youth club to go to that is run by the church.

October 3ʳᵈ

Bills last day at the nursery school. Tomorrow he starts at the pre-school. He has a pair of black trousers, a white polo shirt and a red jumper.

At the moment he is so excited to be starting big school.

October 5ᵗʰ
HAPPY BIRTHDAY MUM

October 6ᵗʰ

Jake is at home today after being sick all night.

This morning I had a phone call from a lady I had never heard from before. She explained that she was from the church that Auntie Eileen went to and she told me that Auntie Eileen had passed away last night. She said that she had suffered a massive stroke and never regained consciousness.

I said that I knew that she had had a blood clot in her leg. "Oh, no." she said all matter of factly, "your Auntie had a brain tumour." "I didn't know that." I said. "No." She replied. "She didn't want to worry you." "That makes two of us," I said. "because I had breast cancer and I didn't want her to worry about me either." We spoke for a bit longer and then she ended the conversation saying that she would be in touch when the funeral had been arranged.

When I had put the phone down I felt very sad, not crying sad but it was a deep sadness. Auntie must of known that she was going to die because she rang me only last week. I felt a deep grief. It was mixed with guilt for not going to see her, for not involving her in my life except via letters. I felt that I had let my Dad down by not looking after her. Realistically, I knew that it was an impossibility to have been able to do that as she lives so far away and my lifestyle. Also recently having cancer would have made it impractical to visit her, as her living in Ilford and me having four young children, some at school, wouldn't work either as the journey, without hitting any traffic would take a least three hours.

Steve came home and I told him the news. I didn't expect him to feel any emotion because he had never met Auntie Eileen but it was as if he just dismissed it, just as if I had told him that I'd had a bowl of soup for lunch that day. I feel really strange.

Lost. Confused.

October 12th

Feeling dizzy again. It is a horrible feeling. I would rather have a pain somewhere. At least pain you can over rule, dizziness is freaky!

Had a telephone from the lady at Aunties church again. She told me that her funeral would be on the 19th at 11o'clock. She said that it would be lovely if I could attend. I said that I would telephone and let her know.

October 19th

Went to the doctors to have my bloods done for the hospital. They couldn't find a vein. The nurse had a go, no luck. She went and got another nurse, she had no luck either. Finally they got the doctor who had two attempts taking blood from my hand. Bingo, blood.

It was the first time that I have gone light headed having blood taken.

I didn't go to Aunties funeral today. I wish I could, but I can't. I'm too tired, not sleepy tired, more of a physical tiredness. One where you just find that your get up and go has got up and gone.

Molly had a football match today. They lost. No surprise there!

Had my appointment at the hospital with the Oncologist. He asked about the dizziness and light headiness. I said that I still suffering from it.

He asked me to stand with my feet together and close my eyes. He then asked me to walk one foot in front of the other. He said that he didn't think that it had gone to my brain but would ask for an MRI scan. I said that the implants were still uncomfortable. He said that he couldn't rule out that the cancer had returned and would ask for another bone scan.

He then said that he would not want to see me until June. I am seeing the surgeon in February. I said that that was a gap of four months? He said yes that was right and that he felt comfortable doing so.

That confused me, if he was giving me scans in case it had returned why was he making the next appointment in a longer time? The two statements conflicted each other. My bloods came back fine. No indications there, the only thing was that I was low on potassium. Eat more bananas.

I went down to the scanning department and they gave me an appointment for next Thursday. I went home feeling nothing.

Maybe I am getting depressed. Everything is becoming too much. I don't want to be part of anything. I don't want to be mum anymore or a wife, but I don't want to die either.

Maybe I need a holiday....on my own?

I need to find me again. The real me is lost.

It is hidden under all the pseudonyms that make up my daily life.

October 22nd

Took Steve a bacon and egg sandwich for his breakfast now that they are back on site in Swindon.

Got more details from the solicitors and they also asked for a preferred moving date.

Steve and I went to see the people that we are buying the house from as we thought that if we had the same moving date that it would speed the process up. They said that they were having hold ups at their end.

October 23rd

Rotten day. Feeling down.

Keep imagining their lives with me not here.

Not very healthy thoughts.

October 24th

Rang the hospital to find out how dangerous the injection I need for the bone scan is to small children. The nurse said that it is fine to be in the same room as them but she doesn't advise you to sit next to them on the sofa and watch a Walt Disney film. Small cuddles are allowed. She also advised that someone else bath them and put them to bed. That was good news. They could stay at home rather than going to Mum and Dads like they did last time. I was relieved as Steve had told me that he didn't want anyone to know that I was having the tests as it would only worry them.

October 27th

I got the children ready for the day. Auntie Jill came over and sat with them so that I could go to the hospital. I got there for my first appointment which was at 9;45. I went to the nuclear medicine department and sat ready for my injection. I explained to the nurse that it was becoming more difficult to extract blood or put anything in me as my veins were not very good anymore, in fact they had had enough. She smiled and had a look.

Yes, she agreed my veins were rubbish. She suggested that I run some hot over the back of my hand so that hopefully the veins would come up a bit better. It worked. She used the smallest needle that they had. It had a tube attached so that she could make sure that it was still in the vein when she was administrating the drug. First she put in some saline and then the drug and after some more saline just to make sure it had all gone in. She put on a plaster and told me to keep massaging my hand to make sure that none of the drug 'leaked' out. As I came out of the room there was a lady waiting to have the same thing done.

The door was open to the room where the scanner is and she got her self in a right old pickle as she was very frightened about what was going to happen. I tried to put her mind at rest but I don't think that I was very convincing.

I had enough time to go home and get changed because the brain scan (M.R.I) letter that I was sent stated that you were not allowed to wear eye make up or any clothing that had metal fastenings and I had my jeans on and mascara. After I had got changed I went back up to the hospital. I was seen straight through because I had had the injection and was a danger to pregnant women and babies.

In the room I saw the nurse filling a syringe with liquid. "Is that for me?" I asked. "Yes." She said. "We give you an injection before your second scan." I explained that my veins were not very good and that they could only use one arm. She said that it was not a problem and that if she could not find a vein then they would call a doctor. She said either way for me not to worry.

They put my handbag in a locker and hung the key up. They walked me into the scanning room. The machine was huge. It had a bench where you laid down and behind your head was a huge thick tunnel that the bench slid into.

They laid me down on the bench and placed two blocks one either side of my head just above my shoulders to keep me still.

They placed a button in my hand in case I needed assistance during the scan and earphones on my ears so that I could listen to some music as they said the machine was a bit loud, finally they placed a grid over my face.

It reminded me of that film, The Man In The Iron Mask. It was very claustrophobic. The mask had a mirror that enabled you to see your feet. It was very disconcerting. I closed my eyes.

The bench moved back into the tunnel. The machine started to whirl and grind.

They started the music. It was chamber music. It reminded me of the music that they play in the chapel of rest. 'I'm not dead yet.' I thought to myself. I maybe soon if the results of this scan are not good though. I imagined the machine slicing pieces of my brain up, like I used to do with Ox Tongue and ham at the delicatessen, my first job. I laid there for what seemed like ages.

A mans voice spoke to me but at the same time the machine started clanging and banging. I took a deep breath. I searched through my memory for my Dad. He was far away today. Was that a bad omen?

The man spoke again. I couldn't understand what he was saying. The machine was making a noise and he had an accent, which didn't help. I opened my eyes, they didn't focus. I could feel myself beginning to panic. I took some deep breathes, don't panic, don't panic, relax, it's not going to hurt you. I was going to squeeze the button, when I began to calm down, I had closed my eyes again.

The machine began to bang, it reminded me of the children walking 'quietly' around upstairs.

I felt the bench move, I opened my eyes, the nurse was standing next to me. She took my arm, she was talking to me but I couldn't hear her.

I felt very vulnerable, I could feel tears filling my eyes. I dared not move. The nurse removed the earphones and handed me a tissue. I asked if I could sit up. She said that I couldn't as it would take longer to reset the machine than the time left for the scan, even though they needed to inject me.

The nurse tries to inject my arm, she couldn't find a vein, she said that she was going to get a doctor.

'No more, I can't cope with any more. If it has gone into my brain how will I cope? How will any of us cope?'

The doctor came into the room. It was the same doctor that had done all my other scans, the ones on my liver and ovaries. She also did the scans on Jake. She gave me a big smile. I felt relief from seeing a friendly face. Tears clouded my vision.

She rubbed my arm. "Don't worry." she said. "I have been watching the scans and I can see absolutely nothing wrong with your scans, they are completely normal and I am going to write to your oncologist saying that. I am not even going to do the last scan. You can go home."

She gave me an understanding nod. I sat up and wiped my eyes. I thanked everyone and went outside.

People were looking at me as I went out. Sadness on their faces for me. If only they knew the half of what I felt. Relief? Happiness? No, anger? Maybe, I'm not sure. My emotions were confusing me I didn't know how I felt. I dialed my Mums number. What was the point? Steve had said not to tell anyone about the scans, so I would have to explain why I was having them first before I could tell her that I was o.k. I disconnected it and telephoned Steve. I knew that he was working a long way away, but I had to speak to someone.

It rang, nobody answered.

Now I was cross. He should have been here.

I should not have gone through that on my own.

That wasn't fair. My phone rang. It was Steve.

The line was bad and I couldn't hear him very well. "The scan was clear." I blubbed. "Told you that there was nothing to worry about." he replied. "You should have been here." I said."It wasn't right I went through it on my own. It wasn't fair." he said that he was sorry but that he had known that it was going to be alright. He asked what time the next scan was and that he would ring me after that to see how it had gone.

I went home to smiles and cuddles from Bill and Fred. Auntie Jill asked how it had gone. I told her that it was the most scary, frightening experience that I had ever been through, and that was true.

I never wanted to go through that ever again!

I made some lunch for Auntie Jill and the boys before getting changed again and going back to the hospital for my bone scan.

I was seen straight away. I took off my shoes and laid down on the bed thing. I had to turn my head to the left and the machine came down really close to my face just like last time.(October 4th 2004)

It was all the same except this time they wanted to do an extra x-ray on the left hand side of my pelvis as they said that it looked like it was crumbling, maybe with arthritis. They also said that the scan was exactly the same as last time which meant........NO CANCER!!!!!!

I was so pleased that I could have cuddled the nurse.

Arthritis? I could live with that. A dodgey pelvis?

No problem.

I'm sure that I was the happiest person alive to be told that at the age of 34 I had an arthritic pelvis!

I went home feeling as if I had been on death row and had been given a reprieve at the eleventh hour!

As I went out of the hospital I felt the sunshine on my face and thanked God for loving me.

I never wanted to go through the mental turmoil of not knowing if the cancer had come back again. It destroys you. It eats you up, takes all your energy and fills your mind every waking moment. It makes you imagine everyones lives if you were not there. It makes you imagine their day to day lives without you in them.

At home Auntie Jill, Bill and Fred had had a lovely morning cutting up card and using stickers, how I wished that my morning had been the same.

Steve rang at half past two and I told him the results of the bone scan. Yet again he proclaimed that he had been right and that there had been nothing to worry about. "They only sent you to have the scans to cover themselves." he said....I hate know-alls. Especially one that I am married to!

Tania Bond

The mind is a very powerful thing. They say mind over matter. The trouble is that you only have to plant a small niggle in your mind and it plays on it. It gets bigger and bigger until it takes up all your daytime thoughts. You always think of the worst scenario possible and then you multiply it until you panic and cannot control it anymore. All it takes someone level headed and a professional in their field to say the right words and the out of control niggle goes away.

October 30th

Had a lovely cozy Sunday. Big roast dinner, lazy afternoon and then helped the children make their pumpkins.

October 31st

Made some banners and decorated the house for Halloween. Molly became a witch and she went to a party at her friends house. Jake became a ghost and Bill became a big pumpkin.

November

November 3rd

Jake went to school for the first time since being poorly. His first day at Dorcan Technological College.

November 4th

Put Taz into the kennels for the weekend as we are going to Hayling Island again for my birthday.

It was a lovely surprise for Jake, Molly, Bill and Fred because Steve had also invited his Mum and Dad, my Mum and Ian and also John and Lucy to come.

The children didn't know anything and their faces were wonderful to see.

The weekend was a total success. Everyone had a fantastic time. The weather was good, the food was delicious, the entertainment was 'top drawer'.

Jake got me 'Elvis's' autograph. My Mum showed of her skills on the dance floor. I had a dance with Dad and Steve kept the bar profits up!

It was the perfect way to celebrate my birthday.

I have the most wonderful husband in the world......sometimes!

November 6th
HAPPY BIRTHDAY ME!!!
What a difference from last year. Even though I am celebrating at the same place the way I feel couldn't be more different. I am so happy. Last year I had all the treatments to go through and now they are all over and are fast becoming a nasty memory that is getting fainter and fainter as the days go by. No looking back. Look forward, be positive Mrs Bond and have a wonderful birthday weekend with your family.

November 7th
We all said our goodbyes and went our separate ways. Collected Taz from the kennels.

November 8th
Steve home from work. He has damaged his ribs.

November 10th
Bill came home from school with a letter. He is going to be a reindeer in the school play!

November 11th
Steve working back in Swindon again.

November 15th
Today is not a good day.
I feel really distant and sad. I keep crying and feel lonely. It is true that you can be in a room full of people and feel alone. I feel full of self pity. I want to run away but I don't know where to go.

November 19th
Had a skip delivered and cleared out the shed and the loft ready for the move. What a load of old junk we have.

November 20th

Bill isn't very well today. He spent the day laying on the sofa. John went to see Bob Dylan at the Brixton Academy.

Today is the anniversary of cousin Sharon. We sent a card to Uncle Johnny. The first year anniversary is the most painful. If someone else remembers it and sends a card I think that it makes it a little bit easier because you know that they haven't been forgotten by everyone.

November 21st

Bill was sick.

November 22nd

Bill was sick again.

Got our moving date 6th December.

November 24th

Molly played football. Amazingly they lost again! It doesn't matter to Molly how many the other team score and they don't. She always smiles.

November 25th

Cold tap won't turn off. Had to ring Steve at work. He came home and turned of the water at the mains. Filled everything we could with water, bath, saucepans and jugs.

The plumber came round and swapped over the tap tops so we have only got cold water. Better than nothing. The plummer is coming back tomorrow to finish of.

November 26th

All mended! Hot and cold running water again.

How we missed it!

Rang mum and invited her, Ian and Woolley (my grandma) for Christmas in our new home. I hope I haven't jinxed it seeing as we haven't moved in there yet?

November 28th

This evening it started to snow. Huge, beautiful flakes. It doesn't matter how old I am I get so excited when I see that it is snowing. I get butterflies in my tummy! I wrapped all the children up and we walked in the dark and in the heavy snow to the library. Steve said that we were mad. But it had to be done. Got home, we were all freezing. Bathed the children in a lovely hot bath and put them to bed.

November 29th

The car has given up, it must be too cold for it. Still snowing.

Got a letter from the genealogists at Oxford, they need some more information about Auntie to carry on their investigations. Will give it to Mum when she comes down on Saturday.

Walked to the Co-op with Fred in the snow.

December

December 1st

Went into town and transferred the money for the new house. No going back now! Raining.

December 2nd

All the monies have cleared. Now it is up to the solicitor.

We all went to the Age Concern Hall to help deliver Christmas boxes to the needy. A big bag of chips from the fish & chip shop helped the deliveries!

Went to see the school near our new house that Molly will be going to. It was lovely, much smaller than the one that she is at but seems friendlier. With her there will be twenty five children in the top year!

December 3rd

My mum has arrived. Lucy also came down to 'help'. She is absolutely rubbish!

December 4th

Borrowed a van from Steve's brother. Packed up shed, garden and the loft.

December 5th

Mum and I packed up the house.

Last night in this house.

This is going to be the beginning of the rest of my life. When I leave this house I will leave the cancer and all that came with it behind in the old house. When I walk into the new house it will be a new page, clean and unblemished, fresh, untarnished. A new me that no one knows the history of. I can reinvent myself, change the way I dress, become more adventurous in my outfits. Take on a new identity.

I don't know whether it is all the water that I have drunk during the chemotherapy and radiotherapy or the treatments themselves but the skin on my face seems to be really nice, smooth and clear.

Chapter 9

December 6th
MOVING DAY!!!!! Chaos!

December 7th
Don't know where anything is. Can't find anything. Want my old house back!

December 8th
Nightmare! Worse than yesterday. I hate not being in control, it makes me panic and become edgy. I need to have routine and everything in its place. Clutter and disarray only confuse me. It makes me become angry and aggressive. I seem to feel like this a lot lately. I don't seem to have a very high tolerance level.

December 9th
My Mum got 'happy' on her red wine, much to the amusement of Jake and Molly.
Steve got lost coming home from the pub. I thought that he was a bit late!

December 11th
First Sunday roast cooked in the new oven. I want my old oven back.

December 12th

Man came to fix the aerial, we now have television.

Mum, Dad, Auntie Jill, me and Fred went to see Bill in his Christmas play as a reindeer. He was the only one not to sing or smile. A proper Bond boy.

December 13th

The children and I have put up all the Christmas decorations and Steve decorated the Christmas tree. Beautiful.

December 15th

Went with Bill to see his new school. He starts the same day as Molly. January 4th. Went to Molly's new school and gave in the registration forms.

December 17th

All the Christmas cooking is finished. Puddings, mince meat and pies and now the cake is finished, all iced. Everyone is getting in the mood. John is so excited, even more than Jake, Molly, Bill and Fred.

December 19th

Bill's last day at school.

They had a Christmas party. Bill thought they had had for him because he was leaving.

I don't think they thought that he was quite that special!

December 20th

Jake and Molly's last day at school.

Molly was crying as I picked her up. Gave her a big hug. Soppy old thing.

December 21st

Steve's last day at work. Everyone is home.

Steves Christmas drink started at 1:30, lunchtime and ended at 10:30pm!

December 24ᵗʰ

My mum, Ian and Woolley arrive. So does Lucy and John. We have got a full house.

Mum and Dad brought over the turkey and some more plates and bits and bobs.

Everyone is so happy and excited. This is just how it should be. We took the children to see

Father Christmas. When asked what he wanted for Christmas Jake replied.

'Nothing I just want to be with my family!' Father Christmas and I looked at each other and asked him to repeat himself, as we thought that we had misheard. I am mystified!

December 25ᵗʰ

MERRY CHRISTMAS!

It was a perfect day! The front room was full of wrapping paper, boxes, presents and people.

Christmas lunch was delicious everyone toasted anything they could think of, Dad made a speech and then we had a concert with us all blowing the whistles that we had in our crackers and following Steve being a conductor. Laugh? Tears were rolling down my face. Simple things make the greatest pleasure.

John left in the afternoon he has gone to Dowies as Vince is having a party tonight.

Mum and Dad went home not long after. Steve and Woolley went to sleep. The perfect Christmas day, just how it should be. Spot on Bondy!

December 26ᵗʰ

Raining, so we played silly games all day.

Lucy went home. Having lunch at her boyfriends.

December 27ᵗʰ

My mum, Ian and Woolley went home. There was thick snow when they arrived home and they had to dig themselves INTO the driveway!

December 31ˢᵗ

I know what I wish for the New Year, but I am not going to jinx it by saying it out aloud!

They say that when your hair comes back it always comes back curly. It is known as chemo curl. I have curls, well at the moment I look like I have got an old womans perm because they are quite close on my head.

In the newspapers there was an article about hair. It said that one of the most famous hair product companies had done some research and found out that there are two types of hair follicles; straight hair grows from straight follicles and curly hair from curly follicles. If that is right how come that before chemotherapy I had straight hair and after it I have got curly hair?

Chapter 10

2006
January

Welcome to 2006!

Everyone has gone back to school and work and life carries on as normal.

Bill and Molly have started at their new schools and have settled down really well.

Jake is just Jake, getting into trouble and mischief.

Our new house is beautiful and huge. The children have got used to having a bedroom each and are sleeping longer in the mornings. The road that we live in is quiet and we no longer live on a bus route, which has made my Mum happy.

The children love the fact that we have a park behind our back fence and it seems so much safer for them. Bliss.

January 7th

Today I am fed up, deep down fed up, dragging you down not having the energy to be bothered with anyone, fed up. I feel so rotten that it is not even worth telling you about it, sort of day.

January 8th

It is even worse today that it was yesterday. What a shit day!

Sunday is supposed to be that day of rest, which it is, as long as you are not a mum. Everyone else gets a lay in and has a lazy day and poor old mum is up making a full English roast with a pudding for lunch and breakfasts in bed for everyone. Maybe it is just me and I am stupid, but, either way I still had a shit day, so because I did, everyone else did as well!

January 11ᵗʰ

Bill had his first lesson of p.e. at school. He had to take shorts and t-shirt to change into. It is so sweet.

January 12ᵗʰ

Today Bill rode his new bike that he got from Mum and Dad for Christmas to school. He rode so slowly that it would have been quicker to walk. Even Fred beat him there!

I am getting awful pains in my stomach. They start from just under my rib cage and go down to my abdomen and around the sides and into my back.

There is also a feeling of pressure in the bottom of my back near the coccyx's. I get the same feeling just before my period each month, but this has stayed the whole time and is beginning to feel horrible.

January 15ᵗʰ

Tonight in bed the pain in my stomach got unbelievable. I couldn't move. It even hurt to breathe. Steve said that it was trapped air and went and got me some settlers. I laid still and sucked the tablets, slowly they began to work.

Steve was right it was trapped air and I soon became much more comfortable.

My Mum and Ian are going on holiday to Tenerife.

February

February 1ˢᵗ

This afternoon Molly had an appointment at the doctors because she had become sore. The doctor examined her and prescribed her some cream.

The doctor also asked how I was. I told her that I had been having pains in my stomach and lower back. She said that it sounded like Irritable Bowel Syndrome and prescribed some tablets to take three times a day.

February 2nd

I feel alive! This morning is beautiful, the world is beautiful and so is everything in it. I have had a smile on my face all day!

How come sometimes I am so happy other times so sad? The difference in my moods are quite dramatic.

February 4th

My Mum and Ian are back from holiday. They are very tired as they had a seven hour delay!

February 13th

This evening we took Taz to the vets. Since we moved she seems to have been losing her hair.

The backs of her back legs are almost bald and the hair on her sides is very thin.

The vet took some skin scrapings and told us to come back for the results.

When we went back she said that there was some good news, Taz didn't have mange.

She said that she thought that she had sensitive skin. The people that had lived in our house before us had had many cats and she thought that Taz was allergic to either the cats or something that they had put down for them. She gave Taz a steroid injection and sent her home with some shampoo that she needed a bath with every other night. She said that we should come back next Monday.

February 14th

Happy Valentines Day.

Card? Flowers? Present?............... Behave.

February 16th

My first appointment with the surgeon this year.

Steve took the afternoon off and Auntie Jill came round to look after the children.

We got there on time, but the clinic was running an hour late, so after a long sit down we were seen.

The man we saw was new to us. He asked me lots of questions that he would of know the answers to if he had looked at my notes or had seen me before.

This didn't help me answer his questions nicely.

He excused himself and went to get the surgeon that had operated on me. He came in and said hello to Steve and myself, he asked how we were and examined me.

He said that he was still pleased with the implants that he had put in and said that it would be alright if they stayed in. But if I wanted, just the bolts could be removed or the other choice was to have the implants removed and the 'jellybean' implants put in, which would give me a more natural shape because they were semi-circular and would 'hang'.

I said that I would like the 'jellybean' implants put in, please.

I showed him that the right hand side implant had become a different shape to the left one, it had become smaller, tighter, harder and that it had a bump/ridge on it.

He said that it had done that because of the radiotherapy. "Did the radiotherapy melt it?" I asked. "No, Mrs Bond, the radiotherapy causes the implant to thicken." he replied, while looking at me over his glasses. Smiles were exchanged.

Well, I thought if the radiotherapy burns your skin, I had visions of the inside being melted and then cooling down again all bumpy and ridged!

He asked if I wanted nipples. I said no, because I had got quite used to not having any.

He examined my breasts again and showed me where there was a small amount of skin that was slightly puckered.

"Ah, but this little but of skin wants to be a nipple." he noted. I looked at him."No, thank you." I replied. "I don't fancy having them because I know that they take some skin from 'down below' to make them. The thought of that makes me say, no, thanks anyway."

"Oh, no." he said looking slightly concerned. "We pucker some of your skin, like so," he said squeezing some skin to make a nipple shape.

"and then we tattoo the skin to resemble a nipple." he said, now looking at me, rather than my front.

"Well, if you are feeling artistic that day you go right ahead." I replied.

I am not sure whether I really want nipples as I have got quite used to not having any.

It has got to be the 'norm' not wearing a bra and not having the line of the clothes that I am wearing distorted by nipples.

But maybe if they are made more boob shape rather than two bowls stuck on my chest I may change my mind. Also if the surgeon has suggested it he must think that it is the right thing to do, and he hasn't been wrong yet, so I think that I will leave it up to him.

The surgeon started to fill out a form for me to be put on the waiting list for day surgery. He said that there was a four month waiting list so I should of just had, or just be about to have the surgery when it was time to see the oncologist in June.

He shook Steve's hand and said that he would see us soon and left the room. We were left with the man we had first seen and finished up the consultation. He told us to go down to the day surgery unit and give in the form. We said our 'good byes' and left.

Down in the day surgery unit I was asked to fill in another form which had my religion, next of kin, allergy details and things like that on.

I gave it back to the lady at the reception desk and she said that a nurse would be along in a minute to go through the procedure of day surgery with us.

I had only just sat down, when we were called through. We sat in a small room and the nurse went through my answers. She also weighed me, asked my height and took my blood pressure.

She explained that if it was a morning operation I would have to be there for 8;00 am and should expect to be going home around 2;00 pm, and if it was an afternoon operation to be there at 2;00 pm and be going home around 8;00pm. She asked if there would be a responsible adult with me for the first 24 hours as the anesthetic makes your co ordination a bit dodgy.

Steve said that he would be there.

She said that that was the only stipulation, oh, and also that you didn't drive yourself home. She said that with her tongue in her cheek, but said that she had to say it as it was surprising what some people did! She asked if we wanted to go on the cancellation list, which gave you a weeks notice, we said that we wanted to. She also said that there was a 24 hour cancellation list if we wanted to go on that as well, we said that we did.

She thanked us for our time and said that they would be in touch. We went home.

February 18th

This morning I woke up and behind my right ear there were two lumps that were really painful. They felt like bites. There were also a couple on my head by my parting.

Have I told you that my hair is now curly and I can now tuck it behind my ears? Cool or what? Well it is to me.

February 19th

HAPPY BIRTHDAY JAKE!!!!

I can't believe that Jake is 12 today. It is true time does fly. It doesn't seem that long ago that we had to dig the car out of the snow so that we could go to the hospital.

I remember holding Jake up to the window to show him the snow and it being so bright that it made him sneeze. The midwives all came round to see him because he was huge. He was over 9lb born. My Dad put his weight up on the board at work and it stayed there for ages because no one had a larger baby. All the clothes we were given, for newborn, were no good. He went straight into 3-6 month size. How he has grown!

Mum and Dad, John, Lucy and all of us had lunch. We had roast pork and birthday cake. A game of pass the parcel, crackers and loads of balloons.

February 20th

Took Taz back to the vets. She is doing fine, if it changes we have to take her back in a months time.

February 22nd

This morning there are also some lumps on the back of my neck, also on the right hand side. I wondered if it was some thing to do with the M.M.R jab that Bill had a couple of weeks ago. I know that the chemotherapy knocks your immune system so maybe I had a mild case of 'mumps'?

I rang the doctors and managed to get an appointment at 10;20. I saw a doctor that I hadn't seen before. He didn't feel my neck and he dismissed my theory of mumps, instead he telephoned the hospital and tried to get hold of my surgeon. He was in surgery but they got hold of one of his S.H.O's who suggested that I made my way down to casualty where he would meet me.

The doctor wrote me a letter to take with me, so with Fred in tow I went and got Bill out of school and we all went down to the casualty department to wait to be seen.

A nurse came and took us through to a cubicle, she put a bracelet on my wrist, took my blood pressure and my temperature, she said that she also wanted to take some blood and asked me to lie down with my arm over the side as this would make it easier for her. I told her that it was diffecult to take blood from me as my veins were not very good.

She had an attempt and gave up saying that if the doctor wanted some taken he would do it himself.

I sat on the trolley with the boys and read them some stories while we waited.

There was an old man in one of the cubicles up from us who wasn't quite there and kept shouting obscenities into the air.

I was glad that Jake and Molly were not there as they would of found it very funny, where as Bill and Fred were too young and the shouting just made then jump a little.

The S.H.O came in to see me, he apologised on the surgeons behalf but said that he was in theatre. He asked for a nurse to be present and examined me. He checked my armpits and breasts. He checked my neck, feeling from the back all around and down to my collar bone. He said that he would be amazed if it was anything to do with the cancer as there was nothing lower than half way up my neck. He said that it was more likely to be a viral infection and that he had seen lumps like this on ladies that had never had cancer. He said that it was always surprising which glands were effected by infections as they don't have a general pattern. He said that if the hadn't gone down in two weeks time to make an appointment with the clinic, but in his opinion it was nothing to worry about. I said thank you very much and FOUR hours later we went home!

February 23rd

Snowing, snowing, snowing.

February 24th

Still snowing. Lumps are still there. Becoming obsessed with feeling them. Jake checks them every morning, I asked him if they have gone down or not as I always think that they haven't or are larger.

March

March 1st

Today is the anniversary of Granddad Bond.

March 2nd

Lumps have gone!! Panic????......Stupid woman, over-reacted again as usual!

Not that there was ever a reason to, in Steve's mind!

March 4th

Everyone has got sore throats and colds again.

Steve and I saw an advert in the Daily Mail just before we moved asking if anyone wanted to emigrate to Australia, New Zealand or Canada.

We sent off and had some forms through. They were waiting at the new house when we arrived.

We filled them out and expressed interest in New Zealand.

They wrote back and said that they thought that we were eligible and gave us more forms to fill out.

We were doing alright until it asked about medical history.......
Cancer. I wasn't going to put it down as I have had the all clear but you

have to have a full medical and chest x-rays and I am sure that it would be written down some where.

Also they ask for any criminal history and I am afraid that Steve hasn't been an angel.

We sent the forms back and they said that Steve wouldn't be a problem as it was quite a while ago.

The problem was me.

They sent a letter that explained the way they work out if cancer is going to be a problem.

It depends if they think that you will be a burden on their national health service (totally different to England where they let you in if you are a burden!).

They wrote that if the cancer was a grade I or II and had less than a 90% chance of re-occurance there wasn't a problem.

They also wrote that breast was better as they do not like lung cancer. This causes a problem as my cancer was a grade III, and at the moment we are waiting to see if that makes a difference. If it does we will just have to wait a couple of years so that I have been clear for three years as they except that as for good.

I would rather do that to be honest as we have just moved to this loverly house and it would be nice to be here a couple of years or at least to see the garden through a season other than winter!

I telephone the man that has been dealing with our case and he seems to think that the difference in the grades of cancer shouldn't make a difference but he cannot give a 100% guarantee.

Steve and I discussed it and have decided that we will wait for a couple of years until the three years clear period so that there will be nothing that will slightly shadow any part of our application. It is strange, but now that we have decided to wait a while it seems that there had been a huge weight lifted off our shoulders.

March 8th

Molly's orthodontist appointment, two minutes inside and she was told that everything was now fine and that they didn't need to see her again and she was signed off. While I was there I made an appointment for Jake as his teeth are wonky.

March 11ᵗʰ

The anniversary of Auntie Dor. I sent Uncle Johnny a card. He telephoned us to say thank you.

March 17ᵗʰ

HAPPY BIRTHDAY JOHN 21 TODAY!!!!!

Made him T- bone steak and chips. He is having a family party on Sunday.

It is also the anniversary of the last chemotherapy session that I had. I didn't know how I would feel but I don't feel anything.

March 18ᵗʰ

I HAD TO CUT MY FRINGE TODAY!

This time last year I was bald and could only dream of having any hair long enough to cut!

March 19ᵗʰ

Today we had a party for John's 21ˢᵗ.

I made a huge ball out of paper-mache and decorated it, inside I filled it with silly things like; trick jokes, sweets, rubber ducks and daft thing like that. Dowie, Vicky, Dad and Lucy came, Mum couldn't as she wasn't feeling well.

We brought John a 12 string guitar and some bits and bobs. We had a roast beef dinner and a big cake and sang him 'Happy Birthday.'

March 23ʳᵈ

Today, me, Bill, Fred and Mum went to the Steam Museum. Trains, loads of trains! We went with the pre-school and had a brilliant day. Fred got his finger stuck in a machine and mum reminisced about her childhood days.

March 29ᵗʰ

Today I saw a beautiful yellow butterfly.

Bill had a Easter bonnet Parade today. Together we had made a huge chicken, so he sat there next to all the other children with little hats on, wearing a huge chicken!

March 30th

HAPPY BIRTHDAY VICKY.

Today I saw a bumble bee.

Did you know that where you have radiotherapy hair doesn't grow? Under my right arm only the top half of the pit grows hair, the bottom half has stayed bald.

Did you also know that after a bath or shower or anytime your armpits are wet, if you have implants in you can make a 'raspberry' noise in your armpit without trying, I find this party trick very embarrassing but Jake thinks that it is 'cool'.

March 31st

Half term begins.

Today I was taken 'On a Cruise Abroad', Steve's words. Or, as other people would say, away for the weekend to the Isle of Wright.

We put Taz into kennels till Monday and set off to Portsmouth to catch the ferry. We didn't tell the children where we were going and their faces were brilliant when they worked out that they were going on a boat.

We stayed in a holiday park, similar to the one that we went to for my birthday, so we had breakfast and tea there. The food was very nice and the children behaved beautifully.

We went to the zoo and saw the lions and tigers and we also went to Blackgang Chine, what a fabulous place!

The weather was dry and not too cold, just very windy!

MY HAIR IS LONG ENOUGH TO TIE BACK IN A PONYTAIL, CAN YOU BELIEVE IT?

April

April 1st

HAPPY BIRTHDAY AUNTIE YVONNE.

April 5th

HAPPY BIRTHDAY STEVE!!!!

Balloons in the shape of animals, a gooey chocolate cake and a roast pork dinner!

A set of knives with his name on for chopping up pheasant and partridge, a book about what you never knew about England and some reproduction newspapers of famous sporting events.

April 6ᵗʰ

Cut the grass for the first time this year, and the first time at our new house.

Bad thoughts and feelings still keep coming into my head.

I can't get rid of the idea that it hasn't gone.

I rang my Mum and spoke to her and as I was talking to her I came to the conclusion that it was because I was never ' really ill'.

It was only a complete fluke that I found the lump, and, in finding it, I was told that I had the worst disease that anyone can be told they have.

So how does that work? You have no symptoms, nothing to make you feel any different than you did yesterday, or last week, or even last year!

So, how can you carry on living your life after having cancer, when, there was nothing to mark that you had ever had it?

Yes, I know that I had an operation and chemotherapy and radiotherapy, but, I never had an 'illness', so, how can your brain and body makes itself better when it was never truly ill?

All I need to do now is answer this question.

My Mum had an appointment for a mammogram today, she was ever so worried. She has only got a month until she has been clear for five years. Fingers crossed! I rang Mum this evening. Everything went fine......

Thank you God.

April 9ᵗʰ

Jake and Molly have gone to spend a couple of days at Mum and Dads.

April 12ᵗʰ

Jake and Molly came home and Bill and Fred went back with Mum and Dad.

April 13ᵗʰ
HAPPY BIRTHDAY AUNTIE SYLVIA.

April 14ᵗʰ
Good Friday.
We have cut down all the large bushes and trees in the garden. Dowie is coming over on Sunday with a lorry to take it all away. The garden looks very bare. I wonder if we have over done it....a bit?

April 15ᵗʰ
As Bill and Fred are away I went out for the evening. Steve and I were up the pub and after last orders we were going to go home when we decided to gate crash the party John was having. We surprised him, but I think that it was a nice surprise. I don't know whether Vince and Vicky approved of 'Uncle Steve' turning up.

April 16ᵗʰ
Easter Sunday.
Dowie came over early with a lorry to take away all the rubbish from the garden. John turned up with Vince and Vicky. Mum and Dad arrived with the boys, who are both very spotty! Chicken Pox.
Everyone was out helping while me and Mum made lunch. Roast Pork.
After lunch the children hunted the eggs in the garden and found all 18 of them and their chocolate ones!

April 18ᵗʰ
Everyone back to school and work.
Good news, my veins are returning! I have one that is on my left hand. That means that my body is returning to normal. I rang my mum and told her the news, Steve? You guessed it, he just gave me the look.

April 26ᵗʰ
Today Fred started school. He went from 12;30-2;30. During this time he and Bill had their photos taken and I said joking that could they airbrush out their spots..........and they said Yes!

Fred seemed to enjoy himself, but I think that it was because he was given some food at snack time.

April 27ᵗʰ

Today was the anniversary of me starting radiotherapy. It was also the first time last year that I went out with out a scarf.

This year my hair is long enough to put up in a pony tail. Last year I could only dream of that. My hair is quite pretty. It is still curly and at the nape of my neck it hangs in sort of ringlets, very girly. I will have to start wearing more dresses.

Bill had his first lunch at school. He thought that it was brilliant.

Fred and I took the car down to Dads as it is due its M.O.T tomorrow. While we were there Fred sat on my lap. He was totally lost on his own without Bill. Bless him.

This evening my Mum got a call from Woolley saying that she didn't feel very well and could Mum go up there to be with her.

My Mum went up to London and found Woolley on the floor....... asleep.

My Mum tried to help Woolley up but they just ended up in a heap, laughing.!

They called the Warden and she said that she was unable to help and an ambulance was called.

My Mum left Woolley at the hospital at 4;00 am.

April 28ᵗʰ

7;00 am. My Mum got a phone call from the hospital, they suggested that she went back there. My Mum rang me to say that Woolley was in hospital. I rang the hospital to see how Woolley was, they put my Mum on the telephone. Woolley had died at 7;05 am.

We were told that Woolley had got up at 7 to go to the bathroom and then, when she was settled she was chatting away to a nurse and then just stopped, mid sentence.

What a perfect way to go.

April 30ᵗʰ

John, Charlotte (Johns girlfriend), Mum and Dad came for lunch today. Charlotte is going to Cyprus for a month, so it was a goodbye lunch and also a chance for her to meet Johns nan and granddad. Yummy roast beef and apple pie.

May

May 1st

Today Steve's back is giving him a lot of pain.

May 2nd

Steve cannot get out of bed .

This morning I had an appointment at the hospital with the genealogist to hopefully be told the family connection of cancers and the chances of Molly getting breast cancer.

I went with Fred. Bill, Jake and Molly were at school. Steve was still in bed with a bad back.

We only waited a small while until we were called in. There was a lady and a student waiting for us. They showed me a family tree and didn't really tell me anything that I didn't already know, except that Auntie Betty died when she was 64 years old. They said that in every cell there is half that comes from the egg and half from the sperm. Therefore, Molly has a 50% chance of getting cancer from me, which in every cell, makes her chances about 25%.

They took some blood from me to find out if I carry the BR1 or BR2 gene. If I do, then her chances of getting cancer higher, but also, Jake, Bill and Fred also have the same % of chance of getting cancer as well.

It didn't frighten me or make me concerned too much as the chances of anyone getting cancer is one in three anyway. So, really they have as much chance of getting cancer as Joe Bloggs down the road.

They said that they would put this meeting in writing and send it to me, they also said that they would let me have the results of the blood test, but they said, it can take several months to come back. They did add that depending on the blood results and there was found to be a certain gene it may be necessary to involve Ashley (my brother) and Darren as they both have children. I went home feeling nothing, as there was nothing to feel!

May 4th

Today Bill is having his lunch at school. It is to get him ready for staying longer when he goes to big school. He is so excited to be taking his lunch, he has been walking around carrying his lunch bag all week!

He came home from school feeling most grown up.

I went into town with Fred and took some of the embroidery that Woolley had done to have it framed. It is so beautiful that it is a shame to keep it in the cupboard.

The man at the gallery said that they would be ready next Thursday.

Next we went to the jewelers. When I went to see Woolley at the hospital, her jewelery had already been removed and my Mum gave me Woolleys wedding rings to wear. They were much too big for me but stayed on under my wedding ring.

I also had an old wrist watch that Woolley used to wear and my granddad, Harry's pocket watch, neither of them worked. The jeweler said that he could mend the two watches and change the size of the rings. I asked if it would be possible to have the rings back for next Thursday as Woolleys funeral was on the Friday. They said that they would have her wedding ring back for me to wear. I said thank you and I would see them next week.

May 5th

Steve has an appointment at the chiropractors this morning.

May 6th

Jake and Molly are spending the day at Longleat and are going to have a brilliant time.

May 8th

Molly is starting her sats today.

May 11th

Went to town and picked up Woolleys ring. It fits perfectly. I can wear it tomorrow. I also went to pick up the embroideries, but there had been a problem with the glass, so I have got to pick them up next week.

May 12th

Molly had to go to school because it was the last day of her sats, so I arranged to pick her up at 10;15, which would give her time to get ready.

We drove up to London for Woolleys funeral.

My Mum had asked me to write something to read in the service.

So I wrote this poem;

Woolley.

A posh address in Mayfair. 'Oow! Everyone exclaimed.

Just behind Oxford Street, minutes from the train.

Through the door, over marble floor into a different world.

Down the stairs and underground to Woolleys secret world.

Plates of sausage rolls, mince pies, empty pastry cases, homemade lemon curd.

Chewy middled meringues, crunchy melt in the mouth.

Everybody knew Woolley, everybody trusted her.

She babysat, house sat and animal sat.

She prepared dinner parties for the rich and famous, film stars and celebrities, lords and ladies.

Summer, Easter, any holiday, off to Woolleys we would go.

All the museums we have visited, obscure ones as well.

Afternoons in Hamleys, Selfridges and Harrods.

Picnics in Green Park, on swings and slides.

Day trips to Cornwall, cold bacon sandwiches, nearly halfway there.

Fish and chips on Southend beach, wrapped in paper, salt and sea.

Crosswords, hours spent, deciphering cryptic clues.

Always a jigsaw puzzle, somewhere to occupy.

Something knitted, not a problem, done in a day or two.

Crochet, little doily cloths, weave your fingers through the threads.

Embroidery, not as often now. Still beautiful to the eye.

A London bus? Don't know the number? Never fear, Woolleys here.

Off my heart, every route, number of stops, what time to depart! Underground, just the same, time and station, Bakerloo, Circle? No surely Central.

Around the world, by boat and plane, train and coach you never wained.

Italy for many years, made strong friend, came back once, your arm in a sling.

Russia next, beautiful, Red Square, you proclaimed, bribed your way with biros and stockings.

Egypt, rode a camel, then fell in the Nile and broke your arm, Cruises, later on in life. Invitation to the Captains table. Relax and indulge.

Pounds and shillings, tenbob notes, ounces, stones, history living. A walking encyclopedia of common knowledge.

Any problem, aliment, query, phone up Woolley, the answer she'll know.

Cuddles, broad shoulders for troubles shared, open arms, there ready and waiting.

Grandma, by blood but never by name.

Woolley we love you, life just isn't the same.

3rd July 1912- 28th April 2006.

It was differcult to do, I stumbled at the beginning and I thought that I wouldn't be able to start again. But, I took a deep breath and remembered that I was doing this for Woolley, not me.

May 15th

Jake has his appointment at the orthodontists. She says that he needs 'train-track' braces.

He will need two teeth out before she fits it. He is not at all impressed.

May 18th

Happy Anniversary Us.

Flowers? Card? Present?

I don't know why I hold my breath for the postman, he never brings me anything nice.

I told Steve that he will miss me when I leave him.

May 21st
Mum and Dads anniversary.

They have invited all of us out to lunch, in total there were seventeen of us. We had a loverly meal in a posh hotel.

So posh there was a man playing a grand piano.

May 30th
HAPPY BIRTHDAY LUCY.

Another pink day!

June

June 2nd
It is a year since my radiotherapy finished. There is only a very faint square on my right hand side. You can only see it if you are looking for it. The only time it is ever uncomfortable is when I am driving and the seatbelt rubs across it.

I still only have hair in the top of my right armpit.

Every time I shave my right armpit I am still very careful because they said that you must avoid any trauma to that arm, I will always have to be careful as I don't want it to swell up.

I still have no feeling on my 'breasts'. Well tell a lie I have around the edges but not across the tops where my nipples used to be.

Also where the weather has been extremely warm, they seem to have become bigger, swollen, making my tops a bit tight across the chest. They are also still very uncomfortable, making some positions in bed no good to sleep in.

I can still feel the muscles in the tops of my arms are not as strong as they used to be and cause me pain when I am doing normal things that involve working with your arms in the air, like washing the windows, hanging up washing and dusting.

I still get days when I feel sick. I still sometimes take some anti-sickness tablets.

I also seem to be getting more bad days than good. I don't think that it is depression as it doesn't last for the whole day, normally it is just for a couple of hours. It still feels physical as well as in my mind. It feels like a heaviness inside me, dragging me down, making everything hard work. It makes me imagine day to day things without me here. I try to imagine how things would be done if I wasn't alive. How the children were and how Steve coped. Writing it down it makes macabre reading because a normal sane person would not even entertain such thoughts and it is not that I am entertaining them, they just seem to enter my head.

June 20th

When I was in the library today I saw a leaflet that was advertising a poetry competition and I thought that I would enter it. I decided to enter the poem that I wrote for Woolley and also send in the one that I wrote for my Dad, which I read at his funeral;

Dad.
If you had a choice between work and fishing, Mackerel wins hands down.
Cod, Sea Bass, Conger, Herring, you always stood your ground.
Sunday starts with cutting the grass, washing the car, a trip to Woolworths.
Afternoon tea, lemon with cakes, a big cooked roast, then wait for Hugh Scully and antique plates.
You held me as I walked down the aisle, a shaking mess with tears in my eyes.
You gave me away, it made you proud. Steve has took over protecting me now.
You were there when Jacob came, held him first, your grandson born.
Molly next, a pigeon pair, Woolley says fair hair they share.
My dad you will forever be, happy not sad my memories.
You have left for a while, not ever you see.
Not gone, just borrowed.
23rd November 1943-22nd November 1999.

I typed them both out and kissed the envelope for good luck.

Lets see how it goes.

I rang the hospital as I haven't heard about my operation and I have got my appointment with the oncologist soon. I got put through to the right department and was told that the waiting list was not four months long, but in fact six months long, I said that the implants were becoming very uncomfortable, the lady I spoke to said that she would ask the surgeon about me.

June 22nd

Today is my appointment at the hospital with the oncologist.

As he called me in he exclaimed. "You have got hair!" It made me smile as I have got so used to having it that I forget that certain people have never seen me with hair before.

He asked me how I was doing and examined me.

He was pleased with what he saw and heard. I told him that I had not heard about my operation date yet. He said that he thought that they looked about as good as I could get, but I told him that they were still very uncomfortable and that the 'bolts' were becoming very sore and I have stopped laying on my left hand side as it hurts too much.

He asked me if I had been tested for HER2 and I said that I hadn't, but when I saw the genealogists they had taken some bloods and that I didn't know whether they were doing the test? He said that he would put me forward as if it came out positive I would be put forward for the Herceptin drug.

We talked about different bits and bobs, he made an appointment for me to see him again in February, as I was leaving I told him that I had written a book that I was hoping to publish and asked him if he would like to read it. He said that he would so I gave it to him and left.

June 26th

Vicky passed her driving test today. She is a clever old thing!

June 28th

There was a message on the telephone from the oncologist. He said that he thought that my book was brilliant and that I should get it printed! He also said that he has lent it out to one of the research nurses and when she had finished with it she would return it to me. He hoped that that would be alright. What a boost! If he thinks that it is alright. I am so chuffed.

Took Fred to the doctors this afternoon as he has some weird spots near his mouth and by his nose. The doctor said that they were a kind of wart that children of his age got. She said that they used to suggest that you pierced them with a needle but now they suggest that they are left alone.

She asked me how I was and I said that my right leg was playing up. I said that sometimes when I was going down the stairs my knee would make me flinch when I went down the first step. I also said that it felt like it was being pushed and pulled from the inside. She asked me to lie on the couch. She lifted my leg and moved it left and right and bent in at the knee. I told her that the bone scan had pointed out that there was some arthritis in my pelvis. She said that it may have gone into my knee, so she said that I should go and have an x-ray of my knee again.

I also asked if I could have some more anti-sickness as I had run out. She gave me a prescription for some.

I also brought some cod liver oil to take every day, it might help.

June 29th

Took Jake back to the orthodontist to have molds made of his teeth ready for his brace. They filled his mouth with this stuff that looked like plaster of paris but thicker, I really felt for him 'cause it made him gag.

July

July 2nd

Had a family BBQ for Bills birthday.

My periods are still not back to how they were. As a woman you have certain tell-tale symptoms that you get every month and you know that your period is on its way. For instance I get a headache a couple of days before hand, I get very grumpy and tired and then just before it I have to eat chocolate. During it I am not hungry and often skip meals, it normally lasts about six days and then I go back to normal, but since having chemotherapy all those signs are muddled up. Sometimes I crave chocolate but nothing else so I skip meals, my period begins (which are much more painful and heavy now) and lasts about three days, during which time I am very tired and then after it has finished I get my headaches! All muddled up. I don't know whether it will ever go back to how it was. But each month they are muddled differently.

July 3rd

HAPPY BIRTHDAY MUM AND WOOLLEY. We have got a birdbath and a rock in the back garden for Woolley, so we said 'Happy Birthday' to her.

July 4th

HAPPY 4th BIRTHDAY BILL.

Bill celebrates his birthday with his pre-school teacher, she gave him a card and they made him a special birthday crown, which he proudly wore home.

I met up with Joy, for lunch and we were having a good old natter, when I asked her if she got 'dark days/bad days/sad days'."Yes!"she exclaimed."I do!"

Here is how we describe these days;

'You physically feel that there is a heavy lump just under your ribs. You feel a great sense of loss, almost like a grief, you feel very unhappy and sad, but you feel too sad to cry. You imagine the day to day life in your family without you in it. You imagine routine things like walking the children to school or sitting down to dinner at the table with your chair empty and life carrying on minus you in it. You don't die, you don't suffer with an illness you just see a world without you in it.'

We came to the conclusion that we should be dead.

Let me explain; Years ago when someone got cancer, they died. There was no cure or treatment that prolonged your life, you got ill and died. Now with medical intervention you live, or last longer because they can prolong your life. We think that although they prolong the physical life they have forgotten the mental life. Your body must know when it gets cancer that it is going to die, so it gets itself ready. But when medicine intervenes the brain is still preparing the body to die, (if you ever see someone who is dying they are almost serene and resigned to the fact that their time is near. You rarely see someone dying of an illness in a panic.) so the 'dark days' we are feeling are the bodies natural clock working its way through the illness preparing the body and mind to except death. But in our case we have beaten nature and survived.

Now we have to reprogram the mind to except that it is not dying and get it to enjoy life again.

After we had had this part of our conversation it felt like such a relief. It made total sense...to us.

Maybe someone should write a paper on it and present it to 'The Lancet' or someone at the Cancer Research. Maybe I will ask them myself.

I wonder if anyone else who has beaten cancer feels the same?

I wonder if it happens to everyone who has had a life threatening illness?

July 7ᵗʰ

It is a year since I got the all clear. They say that once you get past the first year, your chances of re-occurrence becomes smaller and smaller.

It hasn't been an easy year, but it was certainly better than last year!

Chapter 11

I received a letter from the poetry competition. They said that although I didn't win it they would like to publish 'Dad' in a book of poems that they are releasing early next year called 'Flight of Fancy'.

Can you believe it, me, a published poet!......

I replied and ordered some copies of the book, also in the envelope was an invitation to write poems for another book called 'The thought that counts'. So these are the ones that I wrote.

Summer Song.

Butterflies flit across the sky, fluttering so close you cross your eyes.

The sun hangs high making you glow, sending warmth from your nose to your toes.

Happiness fills you to your soul, summer lifts the gloom away.

Flowers sway in scented air, filling life with calm and serenity.

Dandelion fairies, catch them and wish, open your hand and blow them away.

Crickets hum the background beat, birds sing, the summer song is complete.

The Homemade Jumper.

"Oh, thank you, it's beautiful. You made it yourself? You clever thing.

All on your own? Without any help? Is it too big? No, I'm sure I will grow.

Do I like the colours? Orange and purple stripes. Just what I would buy.

What dropped stitches? No, I can't see them. Oh, yes, never mind no one else will notice.

Try it on? See, it's not that big, I can roll up the sleeves.

A polar neck in the summer? I thought that. No, it's not too hot and itchy.

Thank you Auntie, I love it."

I will have to see if they like these poems.

Maybe I have found my niche, maybe I survived to become a writer.

The results of the x-ray from my leg and pelvis showed no change, so the pain and discomfort is muscular. I think that it is psychosomatic because as soon as the doctor told me that it was nothing serious the pain seemed to go away.

I hardly have any dark days since Joy and I worked out why you have them. Self help at its best. Joy has less as well!

I had a letter from the oncology department in Oxford to say that I was not eligible to be tested for HER2 because I was diagnosed before October 2005, but if I wanted to go ahead I would have to pay myself. I am not going to because Herceptin is most effective if taken straight after treatments and I finished my treatments over a year ago, so it wouldn't be working with full benefit now anyway.

I weight 8st 10lbs now and I am happy.

I didn't take up the job offer. Too much happened after the interview for me to be able to except. In fact I forgot all about it if I am honest.

Another Year. What will it hold? The future is unknown.

I have received a reply from the second poetry competition and they chose 'The Homemade Jumper' and want to publish it in the book 'The Thought that Counts.' Can you believe it? Me, having two poems published. That makes me a published poet! How impressive is that if I have to write my occupation on something?

I received another letter from the hospital in Oxford, from the Department of Clinical Genetics and it explained that they had not yet tested my blood for the BRAC genes, but they had instigated the testing to be done and that I would be told the results as they are known. If they are positive and do carry the BRAC gene, then the test will also be made available to my children and also to Ashley, my brother and his children and also to Darren, my cousin and his child.

I also received a letter from the Great Western Hospital which had the date for me to have my final operation. At last the final piece to the cancer jigsaw, once this operation is done the puzzle will be complete and it can be packed away to gather dust and be forgotten!

SEPTEMBER

September 16th

This afternoon we were invited to a family party on Steve's mums side of the family. Her sister in law was 60, so they arranged a surprise party for her. Everyone was there. I wore a new dress that I had brought specially, which my mum and I had altered. When I left home I felt brilliant, but when I saw everyone else I felt like a 'country bumpkin'. I have no self confidence, even when Steve tells me that I look beautiful and I look in the mirror and agree, it all disappears when I am in the company of other women. I always wish there was a corner that I could sit in and not be seen.

September 22nd

One week to go until my operation. When I received my letter I was so excited that it was going to happen. I had been waiting so long, the implants are still playing up, making it uncomfortable to lie on my sides sometimes and hurting when I move. I should be really looking forward to it... But now I am just apprehensive. I remember what the original operation felt like after. I remember the pain and discomfort and the strange thing now is that this time they are going to do it as day surgery!

I am to go in at 12 o'clock and they say that I will be home for tea! How can that be? It is making me feel really uneasy. I looked at the clock at 2pm and thought 'they will be cutting me up this time next week.'

September 23rd

HAPPY BIRTHDAY AUNTIE EILEEN.

Today I have this constant dread that I am not going to wake up from the operation. I can't seem to shake it of. I can see it as an out of body experience where I am in the operating room standing next to the table seeing them trying to save me. I can see life at home after without me as well.

September 25th

We are supposed to be having a family portrait done with Steve's mum and dad and his brothers this evening. I really don't want to do it. How can I smile and act like a member of the happy family when I have got myself in such a pickle about Friday?

I should have spoken up and said was it possible to postpone it until I had had surgery, but, I didn't.

We got to the place where the photos were to be taken and I just couldn't do it. I panicked. Steve was so cross with me. His dad wouldn't look at me and his mum just look so disappointed. I just wanted to be at home. Safe. I want to forget about today.

When we got home I was furious with Steve, why didn't he see it from my point? Why couldn't anyone see it from my point of view? If it had been someone else I would have asked if they were fine about it or if they wanted it done at a latter stage, or was it me making this operation a bigger deal than it really was?

All I knew was that I was getting the same feelings that I had when I had the first operation two years ago, when they were removing the cancer. What if as they were doing this one they found some more? My life was in turmoil again and everyone else was treating it as a normal day!

The trouble is, no-one is telepathic and I don't make myself and my feelings known to people especially Steve, then I get frustrated and angry with everyone, especially Steve and cause a mountain out of a mole hill, make everyone cross and confused by my reaction, when just saying how I felt would be so much easier in hindsight. I don't know why I can't just do it! It sounds so simple but I find it so hard to do. Steve doesn't. If he has a problem or something is bothering him, he just says what it is. I wish that I could be like him.

After a chat Steve understood how I felt and said that I should of made myself understood more. I just feel extremely embarrassed and ashamed by my behaviour. I don't think that I can face his mum and dad again.

September 27th

Picked my mum up from the coach station this afternoon. The children have been a nightmare waiting for grandma to arrive! They get so excited!

I think that I dwell too much on the bad days that I have and the bad feelings. I had a chat with my doctor and she suggested counselling, group therapy or anti-depressants. But, what use would they be? If I had the tablets they would only suppress the feelings and then when I came off the tablets all the feelings would come back, wouldn't they? Talking to someone may help, it does when Joy and I chat, but that seems only temporary as well. Group therapy? I don't think so. I am not the sort of person that can sit with a load of other people and express my feelings out aloud. When I spoke to Steve he said that was what he was for, to talk about my feelings and sort out any problems, he said that was what married people did, discuss things. He also said that he thought that I wasn't having as many down days as I was and that the good days were getting better. Maybe my problem is that I am concentrating on the wrong days. Maybe I should be writing down how good some days were rather than saying, today I felt down and sad, I should be saying, today was fantastic, had a brilliant time with the children, playing and drawing and reading stories. I should recall smiling and laughing rather than when I feel quiet and withdrawn.

As usual I should have told Steve, because as I will never except….. he is always right!

September 28th

HAPPY BIRTHDAY AUNTIE JILL.

My mum came with us when we took Auntie Jill her present and cards.

There was an article in the weekend magazine that comes with the Sunday paper, where people send in questions about their health. There was one about a person who had pigmentation patches on their cheeks and forehead, they said that a dermatologist had said that they were 'melasma.' I kept reading the article and it went on to say that the patches are brown to tan in colour and can appear on the cheeks, chin, forehead, temples, back and other parts of the body. It listed many ways that they can form; deficiencies in vitamins B12 and iron, pregnancy, contraceptive drugs. Ones on the temple and cheeks are associated with alcoholism and cirrhosis, liver diseases, and some medications; sleep enhancers, epileptic and chemotherapy drugs. It made me think. On my temple, the right hand side I have two patches that look like liver spots. I had just put it down to part of maturing,(sounds better than getting old) but, now I have read this I know that it could have been from the chemotherapy. It is strange that during the treatment I was getting dry hands, which was caused by the drugs, the nurse said that alcoholics also suffered from it. Now, these pigment patches can also be caused by chemotherapy drugs and alcohol abuse. Both seem to be connected in their effect on the body!

September 29th

Today I have my operation we have to be at the hospital at 12 o'clock.

Steve and I went and did a bit of shopping and got his hair cut, then we went home and said goodbye to the boys and my mum, picked up my bag and went to the hospital.

We parked and went up to the first floor and into the day surgery unit.

We walked down the corridor and came to a halt, there was a huge queue! It was made up of loads of people lined up, all of them holding their bags. It looked like a scene from a third world country, not England! It resembled a cattle market. I was in two minds to turn around and go home......if I hadn't wanted the operation so much I would have gone.

We booked in and were told to go and sit down, there was nowhere to sit. Some people were called in and we finally sat down.

I was called through and had my blood pressure and weight taken, I was asked if I took any medication, if I had any false teeth, legs or anything else. I was given a bracelet with my name and hospital number and told to wait back in the waiting room. I was then seen by the anaesthetist and answered questions about previous operations and if I had trouble with anaesthetic.

Finally, I was called in by the surgeon. He asked me to take of my top and he drew on me where he was going to cut, he marked round my breasts as they change shape when you lie down and then he drew a line under each one from the outside to about an inch and a half in. He said that he would remove the expanders and replace them with implants through this cut. He noticed that some of the scar from the previous operation had left a larger scar than it should have, so he said that he would re-do that bit. I didn't mention nipples and neither did. I asked him when he thought that I would be going in and he said that it should be about 2;30.

Again I went back into the waiting room. It was 1;30. A nurse came and asked me to get ready. I went into a cubicle and put on a hospital gown, my dressing gown and my slippers, put my clothes in a locker and went in and sat down again to wait, another nurse came round and gave me a pre-med.

The lady that was having her operation before me went in. Then she came out again and went into a little room at the side of where we were. Nurses kept going in to see her. Steve thought that she had changed her mind about having her operation. He said that they were going to make us wait until they had changed her mind and she had had her operation. "They should just leave her and get on with the next person." He said.

We all carried on waiting. The room slowly cleared as people went in for their operations and their husbands and wives went home to wait for the calls to come and collect them.

At 3;30 we were told by a nurse that the surgeon had been called away for an emergency operation at 2;00 and as yet had not returned. That is why the lady had come back, it wasn't that she had changed her mind!

At 4;00 the lady who should have gone down at 2;00 was called in.

At 5;15 the surgeon came into the waiting room and called me into a room. He apologised and said that he was unable to do my operation today as the theatre manager had said that they wanted no more operations done after 5 o'clock.

He said that the emergency operation had taken longer than anticipated and that he would try and see if he could arrange for my operation to be done on Tuesday.

Disappointed, and drawn on I went and got dressed again, feeling very flat we went home.

I feel very strange, empty, I don't feel anything really, an anticlimax, all my emotions were ready for me to have my operation and to feel discomfort and pain and they had to disappear and decide what we were going to have for tea.

I went upstairs and washed off all the drawings in my chest.

Tea, what are we going to have for tea?

Maybe, lets have a drink and a sit down and get ourselves together?

I am finding that I cannot just switch off and carry on as if nothing has happened. I can't just think, never mind and turn on the oven and lay the table. Maybe I think too much? My trouble is that I don't 'go with the flow', I work myself up ready for the job in hand and when that doesn't happen, I don't know how to react. So, I have a go at Steve and blame him, after all, him being a man, it is always his fault!

September 30th

This morning I recognised an envelope in the post. It was from the poetry competition company!........I shouted up to my mum as I opened the envelope.

I was right it did contain a copy of a front cover of a book! Congratulations! Mrs Bond. Your poem, 'The Homemade Jumper' has been chosen to be published in our new book of poetry; 'The Thought That Counts.'

I was knocked for six! They liked another one of my poems! I now have two poems published in books that are available world wide!

I rang Steve, John answered the telephone and he was really pleased, he then handed the telephone to Steve and told him, "Oh, that's good Love." He said....He manages to flatten my mood with a few words every time. I should have got used to the fact that he doesn't do 'excited' by now, but I haven't.

Wow, me a double published poet!

The letter also invited me to enter a new competition asking for poetry themed 'Local Areas'. I will have to think about this.

OCTOBER

October 1st

HAPPY 3rd BIRTHDAY FRED.

Scooby-Doo cake and balloons, lots of fun, mum and dad popped over in the morning.

Lucy came down for the day….. Disaster her head-gasket went on the motorway and Steve had to go and fetch her, they managed to get her car to the motorway service station and dad went later to collect it. We ended up taking her home later in the evening. But Fred had a lovely day, John and Charlotte came for lunch and we spent the afternoon playing with Fred's new toys.

October 2nd

Rang the hospital, the lady that arranges the surgeons operations is on holiday until next Monday, but the lady that I spoke to said that she was aware of me and that the surgeon himself had pencilled me in for my operation on the 17th October. She said that there would be a letter in the post confirming this. I thanked her very much.

I am not very patient with the children. Steve has noticed it and has started telling me so. I am shouting and getting angry with them a lot more than I used to. Things do tend to get on top of me. I find that certain jobs around the house and other day to day things are very important to me and need to be done that day and not be left. Steve says that there are seven days in the week and things can always be done tomorrow. But I have to do them today, it is necessary for them to be done, even if it is to the detriment of the family. I have become obsessed with the windows, they need to be cleaned, the garden, it needs to be dug over and tidied up. They are not really important, but, to me they need doing and I have not got time between all the other things that need to be done and looking after the children and Steve to do them, so they are playing on my mind and making me an ugly monster because I cannot let unimportant, insignificant nothing jobs take over.

Maybe I am still having to prove to myself that I can cope?

October 3rd

Everyone has the dentist.

My mum has gone home back she will be back on the 16th.

October 5th

HAPPY 70th BIRTHDAY MUM.

Jake and Molly have half day and don't go back to school until Tuesday because of Teacher training and opening evenings.

Received a letter from the hospital, confirming my new operation date as the 17th October, I telephoned and said that I would like to except, thank you.

Today is also the first anniversary of Auntie Eileen.

I seem much more emotional than I used to be. New babies, good news, some crimes reported in the newspaper, the children being happy, nature and loads of other things all bring a lump to my throat and a tear to my eye. I never used to be like that. People used to say that I was cold hearted as I didn't show emotion, but now I show too much!

October 8th

My old friend Vicky has had her first child, a boy 6lb 13oz. No name yet. I am so pleased, this baby has been wanted so much.

October 10th

Jake had his appointment at the orthodontist. She placed elastic bands in between his back teeth so that it would be easier to attach the back brace. She has changed his appointment and we will see her again on Thursday.

October 11th

Steve has an appointment with the chiropractor. She says that his back is the best that it has ever been.

October 12th

Jake has the back piece of his brace attached this morning and new coloured elastic bands added.(Jade and white!)

Bill was at school for the whole day today as they had their Harvest Festival. He didn't come home till 3;10.

October 16th

My mum has come down again. Lets hope that this isn't a wasted trip as well. We don't mind cause we love her coming, but I think Ian feels abandoned.

I have thought of a poem for the 'Local Poem Competition.'
It is called 'Swindon'.

Swindon, Swine Dun, the Windy City,
Once Brunels kingdom of steam and railways.
The Front Garden where wildlife roamed,
Flowers, shrubs and butterflies. Jewels, the land adorned.
Now concrete trees and tarmac grass,
Rain fall must follow man-made paths.
Change the landscape with bricks and mortar,
Destroy our nature, erase our past.
A bypass rises, shadowing where woodland stood.
The horizon is blurred, landmark hills distorted.
Artificial light tricks night into day.
Progress, it is said, but, in who's eyes?

CHAPTER 12

October 17th

Lets have another go. Steve and I got to the hospital at 8 o'clock and went back to the day surgery unit. Today there were not as many people.

The lady that was supposed to have her operation after me last week was there. I was second on the list today.

I saw the nurse and the anaesthetist, just the same as last time and then I saw the surgeon again. "Lets hope that we have more luck this time." He said.

Fingers crossed!

He drew all over me again and he said that it would not be long as the list had changed and I was now first.

I went back into the waiting room and told Steve. He didn't seem convinced. We waited and the other people started going in for their operations when the surgeon came out and asked that Steve and I joined him in an adjoining room.

"I'm sorry but the lady that knows the whereabouts of your implants isn't in the hospital yet, we are going to have to postpone your operation until she comes in."

He said that he was very sorry and on Monday had asked the implants whereabouts and had been assured that they were in the hospital. He said that as soon as they had them, they would operate. We thanked him and went back and sat down.

The gloom and a feeling of déjà vu started to fall on us. Would I ever get my new boobs?

At 10;00 some of the nurses gathered near the board that had all the lists on and we heard them mention my name. One of the nurses came over and explained that the implants were not here and that they should be arriving at 11;30... We decided not to hold our breath.

At 11;30 they called my name. I was going in! They double checked my wrist bracelet and asked if I needed the toilet then I walked with a nurse to the operating theatre.

How weird, walking along corridors and through doors to your own operation, while chatting with a nurse.

Once there I was asked my date of birth and name and asked to lay down on a trolley. I said that my veins were not very good so they suggested that I kept my hands under the blankets while we chatted for a while and waited for the anaesthetist.

The surgeon came in and asked if there was anything that I wanted to say. I said that I would like the left one up a bit so that it was the same level as the right one. He said that he would do his best.

The anaesthetist arrived and they put a cannular in to my left hand and asked me to breathe some oxygen from a mask....................................

I could hear someone persistently calling my name. 'Tania, Tania, Tania.' I tried to open my eyes, but I couldn't, they would not stay open. I felt really woozy, my head felt like I had had too much to drink.

They wheeled me into a ward where there were other people all in different stages of recovery. I sat myself up and my head began to clear. I felt a bit sick so the nurse put some anti-sickness into the cannular in my hand. I noticed that I had another cannular in just by my wrist. It was for morphine. She said that I had been given some during the operation and that was why I was feeling the way that I was. She asked if I was ready for some tea and toast, I said Yes.

I didn't have jam on it only a scrapping of butter, I drank my tea and began to feel much better.

The nurse asked if I was ready to get up and she helped me with my dressing gown. I felt ready until I started walking and then I was swaying and wobbling all over the place. I held onto the nurse and we walked into the final recovery room.

The nurse rang Steve and said that I was ready to go home.

When Steve arrived I went and got dressed. As I lifted my arms to put on my t-shirt one of the wounds opened up and started to bleed. I had to call one of the nurses and she put a new dressing on. She also took out the cannulars. The one in my hand also decided to bleed.

We went back in and I sat with Steve, the nurse sat down and went through some pain killers that I was to take home and a letter that needed to be given to my doctor, she said that I should keep the dressings dry for two days and then wash them off in the shower and that the stitches were dissolvable and they would go in about two weeks time, she said that an appointment would be made for me to see the surgeon in two months time. Steve said that it would be in the week before Christmas. Then she said that I could go home! It was that quick! It was 4 o'clock!

I got home and said 'hello' to everyone and then got myself into bed. My mum brought me up some sausage and mash, I ate some but I have got a really sore throat.

I looked down my top, my boobs look brilliant.

I am a bit uncomfortable but it doesn't hurt. I am so sleepy.

October 18th

This morning my throat is still sore, maybe they were a bit rough with the tube that they put down my throat? It is a bit diffcult to sit up, but it still doesn't hurt. I am very tired and don't feel well enough to get up. So I am going to stay in bed all day, dozing and being waited on.

I can stretch my arms above my head and it only slightly pulls. I still keep thinking that I should feel like I did after my first operation, but I don't, I almost feel like I haven't had any surgery.

I have noticed that the left implant makes a gurgling noise when I move. I don't know if only I can hear it, like when you can hear your heart beat in your ear or if it is loud enough for someone else to hear.

I keep admiring my new boobs, they are super. I have noticed that the surgeon cut me where the 'bolts' were, as well as under the breasts as he said he would.

Never mind they are still great!

I feel a bit sick, but I think that it is because I haven't had much to eat.

Keep nodding off.

October 19th

This morning I got up as normal, I feel normal, I don't even ache, my throat is still sore, but not as bad as it was.

Washed and cleaned my teeth and I was just washing my hair over the bath when my mum came in and told me off. She finished my hair and I got dressed.

Between us we got all the children of to school, then my mum cut my hair.

The left implant is still making that noise when I use my left arm so I though that I would just ring the hospital and ask if it was alright, maybe there was just a bit of air trapped?

I spoke to the nurse on the Day Surgery Unit and she said that she would ask the surgeon and get back to me, so I left my phone number and hospital number with her. About an hour later she rang back and said that the surgeon would like to see me in clinic this afternoon at 2;15.

My mum dropped me of at the hospital and I went up to Wren Unit. I was the first in and told the surgeon what was happening. He had a look at the implants and was curious as to the noise. He asked for a stethoscope, the nurse went of, while she was gone I asked him why he has cut me where the 'bolts' were. He said that they had been larger and more differcult to remove. He said that looking at the surgery he thought that it would be better to keep them dry for another three days and then wash off the dressings.

While the nurse was out I asked the surgeon where the implants had been kept as it has taken a long time for them to retrieve them on Tuesday.

He said that they are kept in a warehouse in Wantage and they were couriered in! You would not think that would you? You assume that the hospital has everything it needs on site.

The nurse came back later and said that she could not find a stethoscope. She asked him why he didn't have one and he said that it was against 'health and safety' as it was not possible to keep them sterile. Good job that the nurse could not find one in Oncology then, because, you don't know who's germs I would have been given!

He said that the noises were nothing to worry about and that the body would absorb anything that shouldn't be there.

I said thank you and that I was sorry to have bothered him. I said that I would see him at the end of December. I also told him how pleased that I was with the implants, that they were brilliant.

He said that he would not be here when I had my appointment as he would be away, but then he asked the nurse to change my appointment to the beginning of December instead. He is such a nice man!

Came home and wrote this, the closing chapter of my book.

We did tell Jake and Molly that I had had breast cancer after I had the all clear. We answered all the questions that they asked and explained as best we could anything that they didn't understand. They had a few tears and they gave me some side-ward glances, but on the whole they seemed to take it all in their stride. As we explained, their grandmother had beaten it and was still alive so really there was nothing to worry about. Life carries on just as it always did.

The Bond family life just suffered a blip and then carried on, and me? I'm still here!

Let me know what you think of my book, or share your experiences with me at;

meimstillhere@hotmail.co.uk or my website

www.freewebs.com/meimstillhere

Thank you.

A percentage of the sales of this book will be going to the research of cancer.

I found this in an old book that Woolley had;

CANCER. Cancer is not a disease in the ordinary sense of the word, that is to say, it is not due to any single cause. Some of the known causes of cancer are as follows:

1) continual irritation: cancer of the tongue or lip is often found in elderly people who have been in the habit of smoking a broken-off clay pipe. The rough edge of the broken pipe stem continually irritates a part of the tongue, and hot tobacco-smoke, pouring on the sore, creates a condition of continual irritation which may lead to cancer;

sometimes, in the process or development before birth a small piece of a particular tissue becomes enclosed by tissue of another kind. This may lead later on in life to development of a cancer. It is even possible for a cell that would have developed into a twin child, to get shut up in the body of another, and to start growing later in life. This kind of cancer is called a teratoma, and may contain hair,bone, or teeth. 3) in the laboratory , cancer may be caused in animals by rubbing coal-tar into a part of the body. Human beings may also get this type of cancer by frequent contact with certain dyes, soot ect; in certain animals, an infectious type of cancer caused by a virus, may be produced. So far as is known, this type does not occur in human being.

There is no reason whatever to believe that cancer is hereditary and it should be realised that far more people are afraid of cancer than ever develop it. Nevertheless, any untoward symptoms should be seen by a doctor, especially if they persist for more than a short time. The following are especially important:

1) hoarseness of the voice, lasting for more than two weeks, and not responding to ordinary treatment:

2) any sore on the body, especially in the mouth, which does not heal in a few day;

3) if a patient who suffers from chronic indigestion begins to find that the pain becomes more constant and does not respond to the usual remedies, if blood appears in the bowel movement, or weight loss occurs, he should report to his doctor at once:

4) in women, any discomfort, pain, or swelling in the breast, any irregular bleeding from the vagina, especially in women over thirty-five, should be immediately dealt with.

It must be remembered, that not only is cancer not incurable, but it is cured, in fact, very often indeed. There should, therefore, be no hesitation in going for treatment, and no foolish prejudices should be allowed to interfere. Finally, it cannot be said too often, that there is no treatment, except that given by doctors and surgeons, which can lead to anything but disaster. No disease is 100 per cent, incurable, because all disease is a fight between an abnormal process, on the one hand, and on the body the other. Sometimes, even in apparently incurable cases, the powers of the body and mind step in and determine to defeat the enemy. "Miracles" of this sort do occur, both at Lourdes and in the consulting room of the good physicians, who can instil hope and faith in his patient. But none of these facts can take away from the absolute necessity of using all the knowledge and power of modern science.

www.ingramcontent.com/pod-product-compliance
Lightning Source LLC
Chambersburg PA
CBHW020911290526
45784CB00002BA/508